RESEARCH METHODOLOGY

RESEARCH METHODOLOGY

Prof. (Dr.) A. Mustafa
M.B.A., M.A. (Eng.), M.A. (Eco.),
M.A. (Hist.), M.A., (Pol.), C.G.T.,
D.G.T., D.P.D., P.G.D.T.,
P.G.D., L.L.A.L., Ph.D.

Director
Sathak Institute of Management Studies
Mohamed Sathak Engineering College,
Kilakarai, Ramnad
Tamil Nadu

A.I.T.B.S.

AITBS PUBLISHERS, INDIA

MEDICAL PUBLISHERS

J-5/6, Krishan Nagar, Delhi-110051 (INDIA)
Phone: 011-40167052, 49067602
E-mail: aitbsindia@gmail.com & aitbsindia@hotmail.com

First Edition : 2010
Second Edition : 2012
Third Edition : 2027

ISBN: 978-81-7473-449-5

Published by:
Virender Kumar Arya for
AITBS Publishers, India
J-5/6, Krishan Nagar, Delhi-110051 (INDIA)
Phone: 011-40167052, 49067602
E-mail: aitbsindia@gmail.com & aitbsindia@hotmail.com

Printed by AITBS, Delhi

Foreword

I am glad that Dr. A. Mustafa (Director, Sathak Institute of Management Studies, Mohamed Sathak Engineering College, Kilakarai, Ramnad District, Tamil Nadu), a dynamic personality in the academic circle, came forward to write up this book. He has done an excellent job in presenting the various methods and procedures of research in a very simple and clear style form. The present book is primarily meant to give proper guidance to the P.G. and the M.Phil., students of Management and other social sciences. Elaborate treatment of statistical measures with illustrations have been given lucidly. This book is written out of 40 years of collegiate teaching experience with the students of C.A.H. College, Sourashtra College, Thiagarajar School of Management, R.V.S. Institute of Management Studies, Madurai Institute of Social Sciences and Mohamed Sathak Engineering College.

This book covers the syllabus of most of the Universities in India. I hope that this book will be useful to the students, research scholars, and as well as teachers who educate their students on Research Methodology.

Dr. N. Namasivayam
M.Com., Ph.D., L.F.I.I., D.C.P.
D.M.I.M., P.G.Dip. in Tax Laws
Prof. and Head, Dept. of Commerce
M.K. University, Madurai-625021

Preface

This book 'Research Methodology' is prescribed as one of the textbooks by the Madurai Kamaraj University. It covers the new syllabus which is based on choice based credit system introduced by the universities in this academic year. Research oreinted topics are vividly stated in simple language with lucidity. Not only the students of U.G. and P.G. courses but also the M.Phil. and Ph.D., scholars will find this book as hallmark of success and an useful text to fulfil their expectations.

— Dr. A. Mustafa

Contents

CHAPTER 1 Introduction

MEANING OF RESEARCH

Research is composed of two words – 're' and 'search', which means to search again, or to search for new facts or to modify older ones in any branch of knowledge. The modern notion of research dates from the seventeenth century, with Francis Bacon (1561-1626). In the 17th century science was still closely coupled with magic and alchemy, so that the birth of the scientific tradition was characterized by a careful desavouer of esoteric revelation on the one hand, and popular and ill-informed notions on the other. Curiously, the inclusion of science in the university curriculum is due to another person by name Bacon. Roger Bacon's (1214-1294) own contribution was the application of geometry to optics, and an encyclopaedia of science. Bacon himself fell into the ancient and common error of imagining that there might be a universal scientific method. He derided Empiricalism, but had overambitious hopes for a new sort of induction.

Research means search for knowledge. Research is a scientific and systematic search for pertinent information on a specific topic. It is an art of scientific investigation. The Advanced Lerner's Dictionary of Current English defines research as 'a careful investigation for inquiry especially through search for new facts in any branch of knowledge'. Research is defined as a careful or critical enquiry or examination in seeking facts or principles; diligent investigation in order to ascertain something (Webster's New International Dictionary).

According to Redman and Mory, Research is systemized effort to gain new knowledge. Some people consider research as a movement, movement from the known to the unknown. It is actually a voyage of discovery.

The search for knowledge through objective and systematic method of finding solution to a problem is research. The systematic approach concerning generalization and the formulation of a theory is also research. Research is an academic activity and as such the term should be used in a technical sense.

Research refers to the systematic method consisting of enunciating the problem, formulating a hypothesis, collecting the facts or data, analyzing the facts and researching certain conclusions either in the form of solutions towards the concerned problem or in certain generalization for some theoretical formulation. Clifford Woody says, "Research comprises defining and redefining problems, formulating hypothesis or suggested solutions; collecting, organizing and evaluating data; making deductions and reaching conclusions; and at last carefully testing the conclusions to determine whether they fit the formulating hypothesis". D. Slessinger and M. Stephenson in the Encyclopaedia of Social Sciences define research as 'the manipulation of things, concepts or symbols for the purpose of generalizing to extend, correct or verify knowledge, whether that knowledge aids in construction of theory or in the practice of an art.'

The Contents of the Concept of Research

(i) Avenue of inquisition
(ii) Well defined field of activity
(iii) A well stated hypothesis
(iv) Capable of being based upon observable data
(v) Scientific techniques of investigation
(vi) Logical Interpretation of results.

OBJECTIVES/IMPORTANCE/SIGNIFICANCE/ROLE OF RESEARCH

The main aim of research is to find out the truth which is hidden and which has not been discovered as yet.

(i) To gain familiarity with a phenomenon or to achieve new insights into it. It is known as **Exploratory or Formulation Research Study.**
(ii) To portray accurately the characteristics of a particular individuals, situation or a group. Such studies are known as **Descriptive Research.**
(iii) To determine the frequency with which something occurs or with which is associated with something else. Such studies are known as **Diagnostic Research.**

(iv) To test a hypothesis of a causal relationship between variables. Studies with this object are known as **Hypothesis Testing Research.**

(v) The research is to conceptualize the terms used in any investigation and to define and explain them.

(vi) Research has its special significance in solving various operational and planning problems of industry and business.

(vii) It helps to build on the existing knowledge around the global environment.

(viii) It inculcates scientific and inductive thinking and it promotes development of logical habits of thinking and organization.

(ix) It helps to put the findings into the context of the national guidelines.

(x) Its aim is to make an original contribution to the existing stock of knowledge and promoting its advancement. It may mean generalization of new theories.

(xi) Research facilitates the decisions of the policy maker. Increased amounts of research make progress possible. Hudson says, 'All progress is born of inquiry. Doubt is often better than overconfidence, for it leads to inquiry, and inquiry leads to invention.'

(xii) Research inculcates scientific and inductive thinking and it promotes the development of logical habits of thinking and organization. It is an outlet for new ideas and insights.

(xiii) Research has gained added importance, both for government and business. The increasingly complex nature of business and government has focused attention on the use of research in solving operational problems and planning problems of business and industry. It promotes the development of new styles and creative work.

(xiv) Research means a source of livelihood, careerism or a way to attain a high position in the social structure.

(xv) It explores the various perceptions of the given field of work.

The role of research in several fields of applied economics, whether related to business or to the economy as a whole, has greatly increased in modern times. Due to complexity in business, the Government has focused attention on the use of research in solving operational problems.

MEANING OF RESEARCH METHODOLOGY AND SCIENTIFIC METHOD

According to Bernard Ostle and Richard W. Mensing, Research is "an inquiry into the nature of, the reasons for, and the consequences of any particular set of circumstances, whether these circumstances are experimentally controlled or recorded just as they occur. Further, research implies that the researcher is interested in more than particular results; he is interested in the repeatability of the results and in their extension to more complicated and general situations." Methodology refers to the orderly way of doing things. Research methodology refers to the methods the researcher uses in performing research operations. All those methods which are used by the researcher during the course of studying his research problems are termed as research methods. Research methodology is a way to systematically solve the research problem. It may be understood as a science how research is done scientifically. Bacon says about endless cycle of moving from observation to hypotheses and back again. This simple notion is the end what has brought about so much scientific progress. William Whewell, inventor of the word 'scientist', inspired countless Ph.D. theses with his hypothetic-deductive method (1837). Karl Pearson writes, 'The scientific method is one and same in the branches (of science) and that method is the method of all logically trained minds... the unity of all sciences consists alone in its methods, not its material; the man who classifies facts of any kind whatever, who sees their mutual relation and describes their sequences, is applying the Scientific Method and is a man of science.' Scientific method is the pursuit of truth as determined by logical considerations. Scientific method implies an objective, logical and systematic method, that is, a method free from personal bias or prejudice, a method to ascertain demonstrable qualities of a phenomena capable of being verified, a method wherein the researcher is guided by the rules of logical reasoning, a method where in the investigation proceeds in an orderly manner and a method that implies internal consistency.

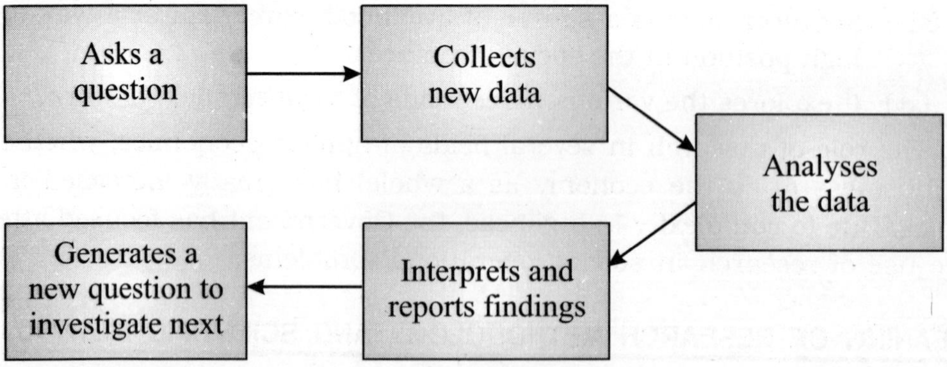

Fig. 1.1: Investigation process.

Statistical Method

The statistical method of drawing inference is mathematical in nature. It not only establishes causal connection between two variables but also tries to establish a mathematical relationship between them. For example, it is not enough to say that poverty causes delinquency. We try to find out a numerical measurement of the extent of this relationship. Statistical methods can at best prove the co-existence or co-variation of two or more variables, they can never prove which is the cause and which one the effect, nor can they prove why a particular factor produces a certain result. The early part of interference is therefore, simiiar to logical methods. The only major difference between the logical and statistical methods is that in case of latter we try to measure the degree of co-variance.

The two methods are not exclusive of each other and for a correct inference both logical and statistical methods should be used. The knowledge of logical methods is essential for correct generalization and its further deduction.

Measure of Central Value

A measure of central tendency is a single value which is used to represent an entire set of data. Measures of central value serve the purpose of summing up the whole distribution into representative figure and this figure contains the gist of the complex group. They afford a basis by reference to which future estimates can be made. They serve as a useful tool for the purpose of comparison of two distributions of series by reducing the series of a common denominator. Measures of central values are most common with the statisticians because these measures help them to reduce the complexity of data and made it comparable. There are three common measures of central value: Mean, Median and Mode. There are three types of means: (i) Arithmetic Mean, (ii) Geometric Mean, and (iii) Harmonic Mean.

According to Croxton and Cowden, 'An average is a single value within the range of data that is used to represent all of the values in the series'.

Arithmetic Mean is most commonly used statistical average in the disciplines such as commerce, management, economics etc. It is the sum of all the values divided by the total numbers. It is least affected by sampling fluctuations. It is useful in further statistical analysis, i.e., useful in the computation of standard deviation, correlation, coefficient of skewness, etc.

Geometric Mean of 'n' positive values, say x_1, x_2, ..., x_n is defined by the positive nth root of their product. It is the nth root of the product of all the observations comprising a group or items of a series. The G.M. is suitable for the computation of percentages and rates of changes, interest and annuities, averages of ratios etc. It is very much used in the calculations of index numbers.

Harmonic Mean is the inverse of the arithmetic mean of the inverse of the values of its various items. It is useful in averaging rates, ratios, and prices. It is preferred for calculating the average rate of increase of profits of a firm or finding average speed at which a journey has been performed.

Median (positional/locational average) is the middle most value in a given values (when arranged either in ascending or descending order, i.e., in an array). For an open-end distribution median gives a more representative value. For the characteristics which are qualitative in nature such as honesty, beauty, intelligence etc., median is the best average.

Mode is the most frequently occurring value. Mode is used in business. For example, when we speak of 'most common wage', We mean modal wage is the usage that the largest number of workers receive. For example, when we talk of most common income, most common size of garment or most common height, the proper measure of central value in these situations is mode. In the case of a shopkeeper who sells shoes, he is interested in knowing the size of shoes which are commonly demanded.

Mode (also a positional average) is the most frequently occurring value. In certain situations mode is the only suitable average, e.g., modal size of shoes, modal wages etc. For the preference of consumers product, the modal preference is considered. For the purpose of selecting a proper average in a statistical analysis, it is essential to examine the nature of the data and the purpose of the enquiry.

Empirical Relation: Mean – Mode = 3 (mean-median).

Quartiles are those values which divide the data into four equal parts. The first (lower) quartile is the value of a variate below which there are 25% of the observations and above which there are 75% of the observations. The second quartile (median) is the value of a variate which divides the distribution into two equal parts. The third (upper) quartile is the value of the variate below which there are 75% observations and above which there are 25% observations.

Percentiles are those values which divide the given data in 100 equal parts. They are 99 in number and denoted by P_1, P_2, ..., P_{99} (P_{50} is the median).

Deciles are those which divide the given data in 10 equal parts. They are 9 in number and denoted by D_1, D_2..., D_9 (D_5 is the median).

Measures of Dispersion are the measures of scatteredness of items around the central values. Dispersion is the second order average. The following are the methods of measuring dispersion:

(i) **Range** is defined as the difference between highest and lowest values of any distribution. If one is interested in getting a quick rather than a very accurate picture of variability one may compute range.

(ii) **Quartile Deviation (Semi-inter-quartile range)** is defined as half of the difference between upper and lower quartiles. It can be found for the distribution with open-end classes. The co-efficient of quartile deviation is of use only in a case where one wants to study the dispersion of items in the middle or the main body of the series.

$$\text{Q.D.} = 2/3 \text{ S.D.}$$

(iii) **Mean (Average) Deviation** is defined as the average of the absolute deviations taken from any central value. It covers all the observations in the distribution and therefore it is a better measure of dispersion than range and quartile deviation. M.D. and its co-efficient are used in statistical studies to enable the significance of an average to be realized, and render the study of central tendency of a series more precise. It throws light on the typicalness of an average. M.D. = 4/5 S.D.

(iv) **Standard Deviation (Root Mean Square Deviation)** is the positive square root of the average of the squares of the deviations of all the observations from arithmetic mean. It overcomes the drawback of mean deviation, i.e., drawback of ignoring the negative signs. It is the most important and widely used measure of dispersion among all the measures of dispersion.

Variance is the square of standard deviation. It is a very important quantity in the analysis of variation.

Modulus is the square root of twice the sum of square of deviation divided by the number of items.

Co-efficient of variation: The co-efficient of standard deviation multiplied by 100 gives the co-efficient of variation.

Correlation: Expresses the relationship or interdependence of two sets of variables upon each other in such a way that the changes in the value of one variable are in sympathy with the changes in the other. It refers to the relationship of variables, e.g., price and demand. According to A.M. Tuttle, 'correlation is an analysis of the covariation between two or more variables'. "When the relationship is of a quantitative nature, the appropriate statistical tool for discovering and measuring the relationship and expressing it in a brief formula is known as correlation." (Craxton and Cowden). It is useful to economists in studying the relationship between variables like price and quantity demanded. It helps to establish relationships between costs, sales, prices, etc., in case of a business. By using correlation analysis, the sampling error can be calculated. It is the basis of the concept of regression and ratio of variation. The coefficient of correlation is a relative measure and we can compare the relationship between variables which are expressed in different units.

Regression: Gives us whether the variables under study are related or not, and the prediction or estimation of the values of dependant variable depending on the independent variable. In the words of M.M. Blair, "Regression analysis is a mathematical measure of the average relationship between two or more variables in terms of the original units of the data".

"Regression and correlation are powerful statistical tools that provide quantitative expressions of the manner of extent to which events are related mathematically. The application of these statistical methods cannot offer proof of the existence of a causal relationship between selected variables. Statistical analyses with these methods can, however, provide valuable information that the analyst can employ to support a judgment concerning the existence of a cause and effect relationship between the variables selected for analysis." – Charles T. Clark and Lawrence L. Schkade.

Association of Attributes: The data relating to honesty, intelligence, deafness, blindness, beauty etc. are qualitative phenomena. The data relating to such phenomenon, in the form of presence or absence of a particular characteristic, are called statistics of attributes. The object of association of it is to measure the degree of relationship between two phenomena, whose size can be measured and where the presence or absence of a particular attribute can be measured. The purpose of the study of association of attributes is to find out whether a given attribute shows association with the other. For example, is there any association between sickness and medicine.

INTER-DISCIPLINARY APPROACH

Inter-disciplinary approach in social science has been advocated by such prominent thinkers as Parsons, Thomson etc., but the credit for giving a concrete shape to this venture goes to Dr. Alexander Goldenweiser, and Howard B. Woolston who made untiring efforts successfully carrying on an energetic campaign for securing the collaboration of the scholars belonging to different social sciences. Their object was to bring to light the interdependence of various social science disciplines like Political Science, Economics, Law, Anthropology, Sociology, Penology and the like, rather than support the claims of these sciences to separate entity and existence as a separate discipline.

1. Definition

Inter-disciplinary approach is a technique of research in which the tools of different sciences are used to find an explanation to the phenomena under the study. It is, thus, a co-operative and co-ordinated research in which the experts of different disciplines pool their knowledge together for the purpose of finding explanation to any problem. Different experts working on the same problem would not constitute an inter-disciplinary approach unless, of course, there is a degree of coordination and co-operation among them. It is a sort of orchestra which consists of a variety of musical instruments apparently playing separately but not totally independent of each other and thus trying to produce a single musical tune.

2. Need for Inter-disciplinary Approach

The need for disciplinary approach is created due to following reasons:

1. According to P.V. Young, "one of the most significant considerations in co-operative research is that it facilitates the study and analysis of the complex web of social, psychological and economic forces intricately inter-woven in modern life." Although different disciplines are separated from each other, they are overlapping on many points. This is because the central focal point for all the sciences is one viz. man. Even physical sciences are studied by man for the sake of man. This is why every physical science has its social or human aspect and every social its scientific aspect. Every new invention gives rise to a number of economic and social problems. Economic growth can not be achieved through economic means alone. It has its own social aspect also and if social factors are not responsive to economic growth the progress is most likely to be held up. This overlapping of the sphere of operation makes different disciplines inter-dependent and thereby creates need for inter-disciplinary approach.
2. No single discipline is complete in itself. Kellogg has rightly pointed out – "Even the scientist is a layman in many fields. If he simply uses the special technique of his own field without under-taking the deeper meaning of scientific method as applied generally he may be as blindly dogmatic as any one in other fields". An economist will be grossly mistaken if he tries to find a solution to economic problems all by himself specially when it involves the aspect that lie in the domain of other disciplines.
3. Inter-disciplinary approach is necessary to avoid the evils of over specialization. Specialization in one particular discipline is essential for healthy growth and progress of that science, but excessive adoration and submissiveness to one's own discipline and specialization in one particular branch of social

science, will only give rise to the narrow minded, dogmatic and egotistic approach. Such an attitude in social sciences can not work well. In natural science, no doubt, we can embrace and adopt such a technique because it is quite possible to isolate certain variables and make a detached study. In social sciences the phenomena does not permit of such an isolation. Its various aspects are so closely inter-mingled that it is neither possible nor reasonable to put an artificial barrier to make the phenomena as falling within the bounds of particular discipline.

4. Co-operative research is also necessary for achieving objectivity. A study through one particular discipline may be highly biased and dogmatic in its approach. The researcher may deliberately or inadvertently try to project his own theories into the phenomena to find a possible explanation rather than making an objective study of the same. Moreover, if the followers of different disciplines arrive at the same conclusion it would serve as a proof of its soundness. Inter-disciplinary approach brings a person out of a particular discipline and takes a more comprehensive view of things. He sees what others have to say about the problem, and this helps him to modify his own views.

Merits of Inter-Disciplinary Approach

1. It helps in the study of the phenomena as a unified whole in all its aspects, and thus helps to avoid the defects of segmental approach. It has thus a very great importance in social therapy and social work.
2. It removes the dangers of over specialization, and helps to remove the bias caused by undue adherence and dogmatic clinging to particular discipline. It has already been pointed out that no single discipline is complete in itself to provide a solution to all problems.
3. It helps is securing objectivity. The researcher has to proceed with wide vision, ready to learn from the other disciplines. This makes him free from biased conclusion.
4. It provides a scope for the study of comparative efficacy of the different disciplines. When the same problem is studied by the experts of different disciplines we can know the degree of similarity and conflict in the approach and the results obtained. This may lead to unification of different disciplines.
5. It creates a feeling of understanding and sympathy among the followers of different disciplines. It helps to remove the dogma and conversation from them and make them more broad minded. It will also help to remove the unnecessary conflict among different disciplines by providing an opportunity to work together on the same problem.

ROLE OF THEORY

Science is popularly defined as an accumulation of systematic knowledge. Such a definition is adequate only to the extent that the words 'systematic' and 'knowledge' are themselves properly defined. Logical argument or systematic theology might otherwise be equated with natural science.

Theory is a tool of science in these ways:

(1) it defines the major orientation of a science, by defining the kinds of data which are to be abstracted;

(2) it offers a conceptual scheme by which the relevant phenomena are systematized, classified, and interrelated;

(3) it summarizes facts into: (a) empirical generalizations and (b) systems of generalizations;

(4) it predicts fact; and

(5) it points to gaps in our knowledge.

On the other hand, facts are also productive of theory, in these ways:

(1) facts help to initial theories;

(2) they lead to the reformulation of existing theory;

(3) they cause the rejection of theories which do not fit the facts;

(4) they change the focus and orientation of theory; and

(5) they clarify and redefine theory.

Theory as Orientation

A major function of a theoretical system is that it narrows the range of facts to be studied. Any phenomena or object may be studied in many different ways. A football, for example, can be investigated within an economic framework, as we ascertain the patterns of demand and supply relating to this object. It may also be the object of chemical research, for it is made up of organic chemicals. It has mass and may be studied as a physical object undergoing different stresses and attaining certain velocities under various conditions. It may also be seen as the center of many sociologically interesting activities - play, communication, group organization etc.

Each science and each specialization within a broader field is an abstract from reality, keeping its attention upon a few aspects of given phenomena rather than upon all aspects. Only thus can the work of science be reduced to manageability. The broad orientation of each field, then, focuses upon a limited range of things while ignoring or making assumptions about others. It is in the light of these considerations that much of nineteenth-century sociology may be understood, for a major task of such masters of theory as Comte, Spencer,

Tonnies, or Simmel was to define the task and object of study for the future science. Theory, then, helps to define which kinds of facts are relevant.

Theory as Conceptualization and Classification

Every science is organized by a structure of concepts, which refer to the major processes and objects to be studied. The relationships between these concepts it are stated in "the facts of science". Such terms make up the specialized vocabulary that the scientist uses. They change as the science develops, for different phenomena come to be of major importance. However, it is clear that if knowledge is to be organized, there must be some system imposed upon the facts which are observable. As a consequence, a major task in any science is the development of systems of classification, a structure of concepts, and an increasingly precise set of definitions for these terms. As the student has probably learned from the history of sociology, much of sociology has been the development of elaborate conceptual schemata. These points to certain phenomena are the most important to be studied and thus helped to organize the facts of social relations. Some of the concepts now used may be mentioned to remind the student that he is already familiar with this function of theory: invasion and succession, marginal man, status and role, class system, socialization, social mobility, and social distance.

Another Task of Theory: Summarizing

A further task which theory performs is to summarize concisely what is already known about the object of study. These summaries may be divided into two simple categories:

(1) empirical generalizations, and

(2) systems of relationships between propositions.

Although the scientists may think of his field as a complex structure of relationships, most of his daily work is concerned with a prior task: the simple addition of data, expressed in empirical generalizations. Entomologists may be studying the habits of social insects in order to summarize these observations in a set of descriptions. The sociologist or social psychologist may gather data on the differences in the child-rearing practices of various classes. The demographer may tabulate births and deaths during a given period in order to ascertain the crude rate of reproduction. These facts are useful and are summarized in simple or complex theoretical relationships.

Summarizing at this level is often not even considered theory and certainly it was going on long before there were scientists. Man's continuing existence depends upon such empirical observations: "objects fall", "wood floats", "strangers are dangerous", etc., are propositions of this kind, embodied in tribal wisdom.

It is clear on the other hand, that such statements go beyond a single observation or a single group of observations. They may become very complex and contain some expression of the conditions under which they are accurate. Furthermore as a body of such summarizing statements develops, it is possible to see relationships between the statements. Hazing of freshman ordination of a minister, ritual circumcision, graduation ceremonies, and baptism are phenomena about which a number of summarizing propositions can be made, but they can also be seen as related to one another: ways by which a group gives a different status to an individual, patterns of ascertaining group control, ceremonial expressions of group unity, etc.

Theorizing on a still larger scale, some may attempt to integrate the major empirical generalization of an era. From time to time in any science, there will be changes in this structure of relationships between propositions. Newton's Principle was such an example, as was Einstein's work on the special theory of relativity. Talcott Parsons has shown in this Structure of Social Action that major shifts of this kind may be traced in the work of Weber, Durkheim, and Pareto as each of them moved from older systems of theory toward a more acceptable system.

It is thorough systems of propositions that many of our common statements must be interpreted. Facts are seen within a frame work rather than in an isolated fashion. Let us look a few examples: "A social is not just the sum of its members". "This is a matrilineal society." "The delinquency rate is higher in slum areas than in middle-class areas." If we study such apparently simple statements more closely, it is clear that behind each of them is a complex series of observations, a set of assumptions about the effect of social factors upon behaviour, and a system of propositions about the way in which groups act. There is an implicit or explicit fact-chain or theory which gives such "simple" statements their full meaning.

Usually, of course, the existence of such theoretical systems is taken for granted, and we do not give them much thought. However, when we wish to communicate with great accuracy or to explain complex ideas, the systems are made explicit. For the scientist, then, it is important that such structures of facts be stated openly. Theoretical clarity demands that the scientist must be more conscious of the thought system being employed than is the average man.

Theory Predicts Facts

If theory summarizes facts and states a general uniformity beyond the immediate observations, it also becomes a prediction of facts. This prediction has several facts. The most obvious is the extrapolation from the known to the unknown. For example, we may observe that in every known case the introduction of Western technology has led to a sharp drop in the death rate and a relatively minor drop in the birth rate of a given nation, at least during the initial phases. Thus, we predict that if Western technology is introduced into a native culture, we shall find this process again taking place. Correspondingly, we predict that in a region where Western technology has already been introduced, we shall find that this process has occurred.

Similarly, we should be surprised to find that delinquency rates in an American slum are lower than in the rest of the city, or that the remarriage rates of divorcees aged 25 to 34 are lower than the marriage rates of single persons at those ages. We have recorded many observations which have led to these generalizations. We expect to find the same patterns in areas for which we now have no data, and we expect to find these patterns in the future.

We expect the same patterns, however, simply because:

(1) We believe we know which force causes these patterns; and

(2) We believe that these factors will be found in the new situations.

This is common-sense way of saying that behind our empirical generalizations is a body of theory. The theories state that under conditions X, Y will be observable. A given theory may be incorrect, but it does make predictions about observations of phenomena. It is a set of directions, stating how certain operations, observations, and calculations are to be made, with a prediction about the outcome. Because sociology as a science is in its infancy, the predictions that can be made are relatively crude. Often we have not identified the casual factors and may make an erroneous prediction. For example, the factors that lead to a high remarriage rate for divorcees in this country may not be found in other countries, and a mechanical prediction from the United States pattern might be incorrect.

Nevertheless, it is clear that theory performs the task of stating what facts are to be expected. This becomes a set of directions to the researcher, telling him what data he should be able to observe.

Theory Points to Gaps in Our Knowledge

Since theory summarizes the known facts and predicts facts which have not yet been observed, it must also point to areas which have not yet been explored.

As noted above, the simple fact of prediction suggests where to test our knowledge. If a theory states a general relationship, such as an inverse correlation between income and fertility, we can see immediately where further facts might be sought. We can break our income classes into smaller groups to see whether fertility might be higher (instead of lower) at the extreme upper income groups; we can ascertain whether this pattern is to be found in rural as in urban areas, or in other countries; or we can study the historical relationship between income and fertility. These are only examples, and the student can work out others suggested by the general propositions.

However, theory also points to gaps of more basic kind. While these gaps are being filled, changes in the conceptual scheme usually occur. It might be noted in addition that "seeing the gap" is very easy once it has been done. An example may be taken from criminology. Although a substantial body of knowledge had been built up concerning criminal behaviour and its causes by the time Sutherland began his researches, most of is related to the more common crimes such as murder, arson, theft, burglary, and so on. It is now possible, with good hindsight, to see that the body of theory dealing with causation was oriented almost exclusively to the crime committed (in the main) by the lower classes. Almost no attention was paid to the crimes committed by the middle classes or more especially, to the crimes which may be labelled "white collar" and which grow out of the usual activities of businessman. Sutherland saw this as a major gap in criminology theory, which pointed to a lack of knowledge about this kind of crime. Soon many other researchers began to investigate this area.

Such a gap would not be visible if our facts were not systematized and organized. As a consequence, we may say that theory does not suggest where our knowledge is deficient. The beginning student must, then, acquaint himself with existing theory. It will then become clearer to him why one research problem seems productive, and another sterile. The formulation of a good question in science is an important step in the development of knowledge. Altering oneself to the gaps in theory and fact will increase the likelihood of formulating good questions.

CHAPTER 2

Social Science Research

DEFINITION OF SOCIAL SCIENCE RESEARCH

Social science is the study relating to human behaviour. Social research is that part of research, which studies human behaviour as a part of society. According to the Intuitionists, social sciences are concerned with the world of human beings, each individual having a volition of his own, reaching to disturbing forces in a unique and complex manner. Social (science) research deals with the social phenomena. It studies behaviour of human beings as members of society, and the feeling, responses, attitudes under different circumstances. It is carried on both for discovering new facts and verification of the old ones. It tries to establish causal connection between various human activities. The individual behaviour may be erratic and capricious but it is possible to predict with remarkable accuracy the group behaviour. It is possible by the Law of Statistical Regularity and the Law of Inertia of Large Numbers. Social science per se began to adopt sampling techniques to measure and to test for reliability and comparison.

Social science research is important in studying social relationships and in seeking answers to various social problems.

According to P.V. Young, Social Research may be defined as a scientific undertaking which by means of logical and systematized techniques aims to discover new facts or verify and test old facts, analyze their sequences, interrelationship and casual explanation which were derived within an appropriate theoretical frame of reference, develop new scientific tools, concepts and theories which would facilitate reliable and valid study of human behaviour. A researcher's primary goal – distant or immediate – is to explore and gain an understanding of human behaviour and social life and thereby gain a greater control overtime.

OBJECTS OF SOCIAL SCIENCE RESEARCH

1. Acquisition of knowledge (academic objects).
2. Utilitarian objects (to understand social life and thereby gain a greater measure of control over social behaviour).
3. The modern social science research seeks to discover and interpret social processes, behaviour patterns, classification of social institutions, persons and groups.

Motivating Factors of Social Science Research

(i) Curiosity about unknown.

(ii) Desire to understand the cause and effect relationship of social problems.

(iii) Appearance of new and unexpected situations.

(iv) Desire to discover new and test old scientific procedures.

Characteristics of Social Science Research

(i) It deals with social phenomena.

(ii) It aims at discovering of new facts.

(iii) It develops new scientific tools and concepts to study human behaviour.

(iv) It is complimentary to other sciences.

(v) It assists in the understanding of evolution of new theories and expansion of knowledge.

(vi) It is an inter-related study.

(vii) It must be objective.

(viii) It takes shelter of controlled experimentation.

SIGNIFICANCE OF RESEARCH FOR SOCIAL SCIENTISTS

Research in social sciences in concerned both with knowledge for its own sake and with knowledge for what it can contribute to practical concerns. Research provides the intellectual satisfaction of knowing a few things just for the sake of knowledge and also has practical utility for the social scientist to know for the sake of being able to do something better or in a more efficient manner.

The emphasis of research to the following persons shows its real significance:

(i) To students, who write M.Phil. or Ph.D. This research may mean careerism or a way to attain a high position in the social structure.

(ii) To professionals, research may mean a source of livelihood.

(iii) To philosophers, research may mean the outlet for new ideas and insights.

(iv) To literary men and women, research may mean the development of new styles and creative work.

(v) To intellectuals research may mean the generalization of new theories.

(vi) Social Science Research has a crucial role to play in guiding social planning.

(vii) It has practical implications for formal and informal types of leadership, patterns of influence and reform in different spheres of society.

(viii) It gives improved techniques to measure new values.

(ix) It has direct implication for social welfare.

(x) It provides solutions to the new problems of the developing countries and offers better suggestions for the old one by understanding the root causes of the problems under given conditions.

Limitations of (Social) Research/Problems Encountered by Researchers

1. Socio-economic and cultural problems and human behaviour are extremely complex. Hence, the researcher is generally confused.
2. It is very **difficult to establish cause and effect relationship** in social sciences.
3. The **problems of concepts** lead to errors and faulty reasoning.
4. The deductions based on past studies and the **techniques used in past may prove useless for the present or future studies.**
5. **The problem of impartiality** is in part a problem of objectivity. Achieving an effective degree of objectivity in a social inquiry is a very difficult task.
6. **Predictability is not possible** because of complexity of social data. Moreover, social behaviour is sufficiently irregular.
7. **Verification** of the results obtained is much **difficult** in social sciences.
8. **Social Sciences face the difficulty** in the use of **experimental method.** Lunberg says, "The social scientist will probably never be able to bring into his laboratory a piece of society there to observe its behaviour in a test tube under varied conditions. He will have to study in wide world."
9. Social Sciences are **less precise** in its findings than the natural sciences.
10. Social research **cannot draw watertight compartments** for each sector of social sciences.
11. **Lack of a scientific training** in the methodology of research.
12. **Want of adequate information.**
13. **There does not exist a code of conduct for researchers** and inter-university and inter-departmental rivalries are also quite common.
14. **Many libraries are not able to get copies of old and new Acts/Rules.**
15. There is also the **difficulty of timely availability of published data** from governments and other agencies.

RESEARCH PROPOSAL

In the research process, preparation of a research proposal is an important step. Institution will approve a project only after a proposal has been submitted. This will provide a basis for the evaluation of the project and give the advisor a basis for assistance during his guidance and a systematic plan of procedure for the researcher to follow. A good research project is likely to result only from a well designed proposal. Hence, initial draft proposal is subject to modification in the light of the analysis by the student and project advisor. A good research must be carefully planned and systematically carried out.

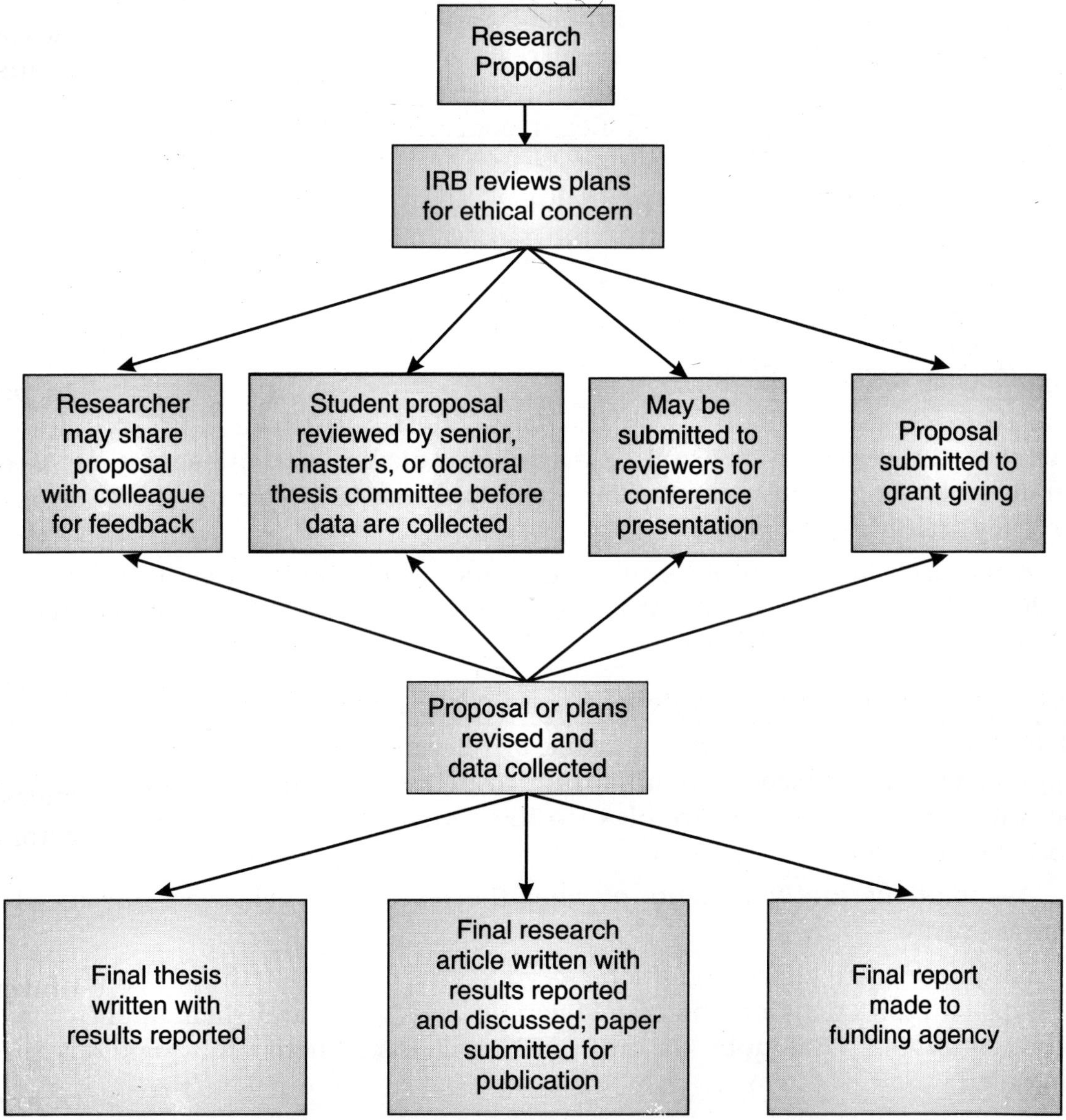

Fig. 2.1: How research proposals aid the development of research ?

The proposal format consists of the following:

Statement of the Problem

This is often a declarative statement but may be in question form. This attempts to focus on a stated goal gives, and direction to the research process. It must be limited enough in scope to make a definite conclusion possible.

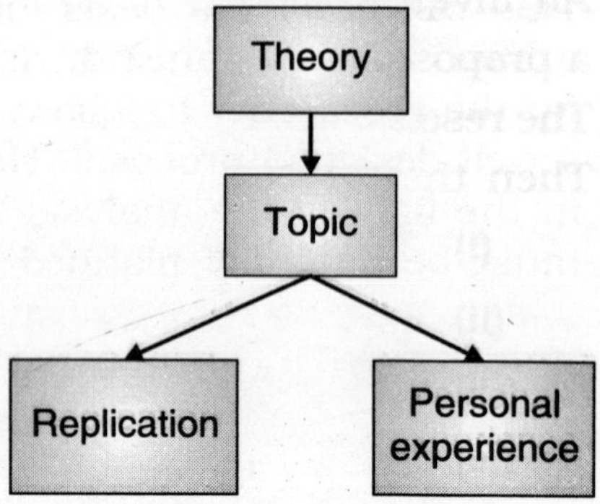

Fig. 2.2: Ways to develop a research topic.

A problem normally implies that a controversy or difference of opinion exists. Problem can be derived from theory, prior research results or personal observation and experience. Frequently, problems are based upon a significant concern. Some examples of problem statements are:

(1) Are children who have had kinder garden experience better prepared for first grade?

(2) Racial segregation may have a damaging effect upon the self-image of minority group children.

Significance of the Problem

The researcher must justify why the time, effort and expense are required to carryout the proposed research. Careful formulation and presentation of the implications or possible applications of knowledge help to give the project an urgency justifying its worth.

A research for data of little ultimate value, would be the result as failure to include this step in the proposal and may well leave the research with a problem without significance.

Definitions, Assumptions, Limitations and Delimitations

Definitions help to establish the frame of reference, with which the researcher approaches the problem. It is important to define all unusual terms that could be misinterpreted. The variables to be considered should be defined in operational terms.

Assumptions are statements of what the researcher believes to be fact but cannot verify.

Limitations are those conditions beyond the control of the researcher that may place restrictions on the conclusions of the study and their application to other situations. **Example:** A data gathering instrument that has not been validated.

Delimitations are the Boundaries of the Study

Components of a Research Proposal

An investigator before getting on to the job of planning a research design for a proposed study, should be clear about what, whom, how and why to observe. The researcher should be clear about how to record and analyze the observations. Then the **following steps are to be followed by the investigator:**

(i) Title of the investigation
(ii) Purpose of the study
(iii) Critical appraisal of review of literature
(iv) Statement of the problem
(v) Scope of investigation
(vi) Objectives of the study
(vii) Conceptualization of the terms used in the investigation
(viii) Variables
(ix) Formulation of hypotheses
(x) Selection of hypotheses
(xi) Data collection
(xii) Analysis of the data
(xiii) Tabulation of the results
(xiv) Interpretation of the results
(xv) Verification of the results
(xvi) Conclusions
(xvii) Suggestions for further research
(xviii) Bibliography
(xix) Summary of the report.

OBJECTIVES

After studying this lesson, you should be able to

- To choose a good research problem.
- To plan carefully and to carryout the research systematically.
- To follow the proper format of the research proposal to suit the funding agency.

Types of Investigation/Enquiry

(i) Open or Confidential

(ii) Original or Repetitive

(iii) Official or Non-official

(iv) Census or Sample.

SOURCES OF PROBLEMS

Sources of Research Problem

- Theory of one's own interest,
- Daily problems,
- Technological changes,
- Unexplored areas, and
- Discussion with supervisor.

The choice of suitable problem is always difficult. Few beginners become aware of a good problem.

The most common experiences in school, college or community lend themselves to investigation and they are more appropriate for a beginner. For example, a student who has moved from Mumbai or Delhi can study about the adjustment problems due to migration; or student living in a flat system or a joint family system can study the effect of crowding on the stress and performance; or a student from Tamil or Telugu or Kannada or Hindu medium at school studying in English medium at the college level can investigate about the problems faced due to the change in medium, effect or academic achievement and the coping strategies.

Classroom lectures, discussions, seminars out-of-class discussions with classmates, other students and professors will suggest many problems for study.

Reading textbooks, research reports, research papers will suggest additional areas of research. A critical evaluation of research article will provide suggestions about the methodology for research.

Consultation with the research advisor or supervisor or guide or a senior professor is most helpful. The research advisor or guide should help students clarify their thinking and develop a manageable problem for research.

Once the scope of the topic or problem is narrowed to make it a potentially researchable problem, then it is easy to determine its importance and feasibility.

Evaluating the Problem

Several searching questions should be raised before finalizing the research problem. Some of them are given below:

(1) Is it possible to conduct the research effectively?

(2) Is the problem significant?

(3) Is the problem a new one?

(4) Is research on the problem feasible?

In addition to these questions, the student researcher should consider the following also:

(a) Am I competent to plan and carryout a study of this type?

(b) Are the data accessible? Will I get the necessary permission from the institutions, or organizations to collect data?

(c) Will I have necessary financial resources to carry on this study?

(d) Will I have enough time to complete the project? Certain projects of a longitudinal type are avoided because of limitations of time.

(e) Will I have courage and determination to pursue the study in spite of some difficulties and social hazards? For example, research problems related to sex education, and other controversial problem areas may pose difficulties to pursue.

Review of Related Literature

Effective Research is based upon past knowledge. This helps to eliminate the duplication of what has been done and provides useful hypotheses and helpful suggestions for significant investigation. It provides evidence that the researcher is familiar with what is already known and what is still unknown and untested.

Citing studies that show substantial agreement and those that seem to present conflicting conclusions, help to sharpen and define understanding of existing knowledge in the problem area and provide a background for the research project and make the reader aware of the status of the issue.

This step is a valuable guide to defining the problem, recognizing its significance, suggesting promising data – gathering devices, appropriate study design, and sources of data.

Methods

This consists of subjects, procedures and data analysis. The subject selection details the population from which the researcher plans to select the sample. The number of subjects desired from the population and how they will be selected are also indicated.

The procedures section describes in detail what will be done, how it will be done, 'what data will be needed, and what data gathering devices will be used.

The information given in the data analysis section should be specific and detailed enough to demonstrate to the reader exactly what is planned. No detail should be left open to question. The information gathered must be presented in the form of tables. Then the data analysis will become easier.

CLASSIFICATION

Once the data is collected and edited, the first task of the statistician is the organization of the figures in such a form that their significance may be appreciated, that comparison with masses of similar data may be felicitated, and further analysis may be possible. But before tabulating the data into different homogeneous classes, it is necessary to sort out the relevant and significant features from the irrelevant and insignificant ones. The process of arranging the data into groups or classes according to resemblances and similarities is technically called classification. According to Secrist, classification is the process of arranging data into sequences and groups according to their common characteristics, or separating them into different but related parts. For example, the data relating to socio-economic enquiry, (family budget data relating to nature, quality and quantity of the commodities consumed by the group of people together with expenditure on different items of consumption) may be classified under the following heads:

1. Food (Cereals, rice, wheat, maize, pulses etc.)
2. Clothing
3. Fuel and Lighting
4. House Rent
5. Miscellaneous (like education, recreation, medical expenses, gifts, newspapers, etc.

Objects of Classification

1. To facilitate comparison.
2. To present facts in a simple form.
3. To bring out relationship.
4. To bring out similarities and dissimilarities.
5. To prepare the basis for tabulation.

Types of Classification

A. Classification on the basis of attributes:

Simple Classification

Manifold Classification.

B. Classification on the basis of class intervals.

TABULATION

A statistical table is an orderly and systematic presentation of numerical data in columns and rows. There are two types of tables: (i) General purpose tables and (ii) Special purpose tables. The tabulation may be done entirely by manual methods or electronic methods. When the tabulation of the data is to be done on computers, all answers must be converted into numeric form adapted to placement on punch cards. Each respondent will be given a card and all information pertaining to him will be entered in this card. If the questionnaire is long, then two or more cards for recording each respondent's answer may be used.

In hand tabulation, we may use the direct tally, the list and tally, the card sort and count methods or strip method. A short description of each method is given below:

(i) **Direct Tally:** If the number of respondents are small say 50 to 60 and the number of tables required are also small, direct tabulation is possible.

(ii) **List and Tally Method:** In this case, a long sheet, double fools cap size or map drawing size is used. On the sheets, as many columns as possible are drawn. On the top of each column, the code number of the question is entered. The responses are entered in the rows.

Table 2.1: Coding Sheet

Columns								Code		
1	0	1	2	3	4	5	6	7	8	9
2	0	1	2	3	4	5	6	7	8	9
3	0	1	2	3	4	5	6	7	8	9
4	0	1	2	3	4	5	6	7	8	9
5	0	1	2	3	4	5	6	7	8	9

This method is easier for small surveys.

(iii) **Card Sort and Count Method:** In this method a thick card with columns printed on the edges is used for each questionnaire. Each column has a number. Therefore, allot code number for each questionnaire/item/variable. Enter the code number of value of the response in the concerned column. Almost 40 columns can be printed on each side. Thus, response for a total of 80 questions/items/variable can be entered on both sides.

Table 2.2: Sorting Card

1	2	3	4	5	6	7
22						8
21						9
20						10
19						11
18	17	16	15	14	13	12

This method facilitates easy sorting out. The cards pertaining to each category in a table are segregated. Then the number of cards in each category is counted and the frequency is ascertained. For sorting out the cards, chalk piece boxes can be used. The main advantage of this method is easy handling. However, if the number of items exceeds 80 this method is not useful.

(iv) **Strip Method:** Long strip of one inch width is used in this method. Each strip has 160 columns printed on each side. Thus, response relating to 320 items can be recorded in strip. The strip can also be folded and made easy for handling. This method is suitable for big projects with large number of items.

1. Method of Tabulation

Hand tabulation is simple involving no technical knowledge or skill. If the number of survey cases is small, say of the order of 100-200 or less, there may be no point in tabulating by machine.

The development of electronic computers has led to tremendous advance in survey analysis. It has led to the use of high-powered multivariate statistical procedures. Most computer installations have large libraries of computer programmes and the research only has to discover how to use the programmes of interest to him.

2. Parts of a Table

(i) The number,
(ii) The Title,
(iii) The Head-note,
(iv) The Captions,
(v) The Body,
(vi) The Sub-head,
(vii) The foot-note, and
(viii) The Source-note.

3. Types of Tables

(i) One-way or simple tabulation,
(ii) Two-way or cross tabulation, and
(iii) High order or multivariate tabulation.

The following tables may be frequency table or response table:

Table 2.3: Frequency Table

Textile Mills in Madurai Earning Profit During 2008-09

Profit (in rupees thousands)	Number of Mills	Percentage
Upto 50	5	12.5
50 to 100	4	10.0
100 to 150	8	20.0
150 to 200	13	32.5
200 to 250	7	17.5
Above 250	3	7.5
Total	40	100.00

Table 2.4: Response Table

Response	Number of Responses	Percentage
Yes	20	40
No	30	60
Total	50	100

Dummy tables to illustrate the tabulations and comparisons that will be needed should be set up before the final research design details are settled. Data from the pilot study may be entered in these tables to indicate whether the anticipated relationship is likely to be found in the study or not.

4. Component of a Table

The different components of a table are:

(i) **Table Number.**

(ii) **Title of the Table:** The title should be clear, brief and self-explanatory.

(iii) **Caption:** Caption refers to column headings. It may consist of one or both column headings. Under a column heading there may be sub-heads.

(iv) **Sub-heads:** Sub-heads are the designations of the rows or row headings. They are at the extreme left. The stubs are usually wider than column headings.

(v) **Body:** The body of the table contains the numerical information. This is the most vital part of the table. Data presented in the body is arranged according to description.

(vi) **Footnotes:** Footnotes are used to give the sources of secondary data.

5. General Rules of Tabulation

(i) All table captions and stubs should be arranged in some systematic order.

(ii) Unit of measurement must be clearly defined.

(iii) Tables should not be overloaded with details.

(iv) The arrangement of the table should be logical.

(v) Abbreviations should be avoided.

(vi) The expression "etc.," is a bad form in a table.

(vii) Do not use ditto marks.

(viii) If any information is not available show this fact by the letters "NA" or by dash (—).

(ix) The table should suit the size of the paper.

BASIC TYPES OF DIAGRAMMES

(i) The histogram,

(ii) the polygon,

(iii) the bar chart,

(iv) the pictograph,

(v) the circle chart,

(vi) the statistical map,

(vii) the scatter diagram, and

(viii) the time series line chart.

Time Schedule

Dividing the project into manageable parts and assigning dates for their completion helps to systematize the study and minimize the natural tendency to procrastinate. Since academic research projects usually involve critical time limitations and definite deadlines for filling the completed report, the planning of procedures with definite date goals is most important.

Sources of Information

(a) ***Using the library:*** The student should become thoroughly acquainted with the university library, the location of its varied facilities and the services it provides. In addition to the traditional card catalogue, many university libraries have computerized their holdings and have placed terminals in various locations for ease of finding books and periodicals. The list of books and periodicals available and the libraries holding these materials can be quickly accessed on a time – sharing computer system available in most libraries.

(b) ***Finding related literature:*** The search for references is an ever-expanding process for each reference may lead to a new list of sources. The investigator, with the help of a librarian, uses key words to let the computer system know which materials are desired. The investigator can then have the titles and abstracts printed either "online" or less expensively, overnight at the computer services facilities. Considering the time that is saved by using a computer search facility, the cost is minimal.

(c) ***Microfiche:*** The development of microfiche has been one of the most significant contributions to library services by providing economy and conveniences of storing and distribution of scholarly materials. A microfiche is a sheet of film that contains micro images or printed materials. Microfiche readers that magnify the micro images to original or large copy size are available at libraries.

A super-microfiche has been developed that contains up to 1000 pages of printed materials on a single 4″ × 6″ transparent card, the equivalent of two or more books. Even more spectacular development is the ultra – microfiche that contains up to 3200 microdots on a single card.

(d) ***Note taking:*** Note will result from speeches and lectures, class discussions, conversation, from solitary meditation, and from reading reference materials. Without a careful, systematic method of note taking, much of what is read is quickly forgotten.

Reading-reference notes have been classified under four principal categories:

(1) ***Quotation:*** The exact words of an author are reproduced, enclosed in quotation marks. It is essential to copy each statement accurately. It is essential to copy and to indicate the exact page reference, so that, the quotations may be properly referenced in the written report.

(2) ***Para phrase:*** The reader restates the author's thoughts in his or her own words.

(3) ***Summary:*** The reader states in condensed form the contents of the article.

(4) ***Evaluation:*** The reader records his or her own reaction, indicating agreement or disagreement or interpreting the point of view of the writer.

A suggested method of taking notes is explained here:

(1) Skim the reference source before taking any notes. Selecting the most significant materials is a skill to be cultivated.

(2) Use 4″ × 6″ index cards. They are easily stored by subject headings and are large enough to include a reasonable amount of material.

(3) File each note card under a definite topic or heading. Place the subject heading at the top of the card for convenient filling.

(4) Include only one topic on a card. This makes organization of notes flexible. If the notes are lengthy, use consecutively numbered cards, and slip a rubber band around them before filling.

(5) Be sure that notes are complete and clearly understandable.

(6) Distinguish clearly between a summary, a direct quotation of the author, a reference to the author's source and an evaluative statement.

(7) Do not plan to recopy or type your notes. Copy your notes carefully the first time.

(8) Keep a supply of note cards with you at all times, so that you can note down ideas that come to you while waiting, riding the bus or listening to a lecture or discussion.

(9) Be careful not to lose your notes. As soon as they are copied, file them in a card index box.

(10) Keep a permanent file of your notes. You may find the same notes useful in a number of courses or in writing a number of reports.

When taking notes, consider the advisability of making photo copies of book and journal pages so that they can be examined more efficiently at home.

REFERENCE AND BIBLIOGRAPHY

The most convenient way to assemble and organize references or a bibliography is by the use of bibliography cards. The card includes the names of the authors, the facts of publication, and the annotation. Placing the information on cards makes it easy to assemble the author's name in the alphabetical order in which they are listed in the bibliography of the report. It is discussed in detail in the succeeding pages in this book.

SUBMITTING A RESEARCH PROPOSAL TO A FUNDING AGENCY

Experienced researchers may submit research proposals to foundations or government agencies to support their research. The request for proposals (RFP) is usually quite specific in the goals and priorities for funding. The RFP also provides guidelines for writing the proposal including a suggested format and sometimes a copy of the guidelines to be used in rating the proposal.

Due to the highly competitive nature of funded research, it is critical that in the proposal author respond carefully to the priorities of the funding agency. Suggestions to Seek Financial Support are given below:

(1) Write the proposal very carefully. Follow the format recommended by the agency in writing the proposal.

(2) Pay attention to stated goals and principles of the foundation or agency. It is important to point out how your study would be relevant to these goals.

(3) State your problem in such a way that the proposal evaluators, who are capable and experienced in judging research proposals but know nothing about your project, will be able to judge its worth and the likelihood of its contribution to a significant area of knowledge.

(4) Indicate how your study will add to or refine present knowledge.

(5) State your hypothesis in both conceptual and operational terms and in both substantive and null form.

(6) Indicate that you are completely familiar with the field of investigation and aware of all recent studies in the problem area.

(7) Indicate how you propose to test your hypotheses describing your research design and the data gathering instruments or procedures that you will use, indicating their known validity and reliability.

(8) Describe your sampling procedure indicating how you will randomly select and randomly assign your subjects or observations.

(9) Indicate the extraneous variables that must be recognized and explain how you propose to minimize their influence.

(10) Explain the statistical procedures that you will employ, indicating any computer application that you will use.

(11) Prepare a budget proposal estimating the funds required.

(12) Provide some tangible evidence of your competence by listing:

- (a) Research project that you have carried out or actively participated in.
- (b) Your scholarly journal articles, including abstracts of your studies.
- (c) Your academic training and other qualifications.

Criteria of Good Research/Characteristics of a Good Research Proposal

- (i) Good research is systematic which is structured with specified steps.
- (ii) Good research is guided by the rules of logical reasoning and logical process.
- (iii) Good research must be replicable (verifiable).
- (iv) It must be empirical.
- (v) Good research is empirical (related to a real situation).

(vi) It must be guided by the rules of logical reasoning and the logical process of induction and deduction (it must be logical).

(vii) **Objectivity:** The objectivity of the procedure may be judged by the degree of agreement between the final scores assigned to different individuals by more than one independent observer. The objectivity of the findings pertains to the methods of collection of data and scoring of the responses.

(viii) **Validity:** A measuring instrument is said to be valid when it measures what it purports to measure.

(ix) **Reliability/consistency:** The investigator should frame his items in such a way that the respondent cannot but give only one genuine response. There are different methods in determining the reliability of the responses given out by a respondent. Some of these methods are using checking items, administering the same test repeatedly, using a series of parallel forms etc.

(x) **Generalization:** The findings of the given area of study should be generalized, without being contaminated by the errors of measurement or sampling errors or any other interfering factors.

The process of formulating and stating the research problem: A research problem refers to some difficulty which a researcher experiences in the context of either a theoretical or practical situation and wants to obtain a solution for the same. The components of a research problem are as under:

(i) There must be an individual or a group which has some difficulty or the problem.

(ii) There must be some objectives to be attained at. If one wants nothing, one cannot have a problem.

(iii) There must be alternative means (or the course of action) for obtaining the objectives one wishes to attain. This means that there must be at least two means available to a researcher. If he has no choice of means, he cannot have a problem.

(iv) There must remain some doubt in the mind of a researcher with regard to the selection of alternatives. This means that research must answer the question concerning the relative efficiency of the possible alternatives.

(v) There must be some environment to which the difficulty pertains.

Thus, a research problem is one which requires a researcher to find out the best solution for the given problem, i.e., to find out by which course of action the objectives can be attained optimally in the context of a given environment. There are several factors which may result in making the problem complicated. For instance the environment may change affecting the efficiencies of the courses of action or the values of the outcomes, the number of alternative courses of action may be very large; persons not involved in making the decisions may be affected by it and react to it favourably or unfavourably and similar other factors.

Scientific inquiry is an undertaking created to the solution of problems. The first step in formulating the research is to make the problem concrete and explicit. A research worker should identify some aspect of the topic which can be formulated into a specific research question which is feasible to investigate with the resources available.

For example, the current research interest is to find out the reasons for the success stories of Japanese industries. The general topic is to study the Japanese management style and their success in global business. There are several aspects of success stories of Japanese industries, viz., administrative, financial, economical, political, sociological, and psychological etc. Similarly, there are several aspects of Japanese management viz., financial, marketing, personnel, technological etc. Clearly it will not be possible to consider all aspects of Japanese management with in the limits of a single study. One of the steps is to select a topic that would yield a task of manageable size. Example is the study of the behavioural characteristics of employees in Japanese industries.

There are two different ways of stating a problem:

1. Posing question/questions and
2. Making declaration statement/statements.

Definition of the Problem: It implies the separation of the problem from the complex of difficulties and needs. It means to put a fence around it, to separate it by careful distinctions from like questions found in related situations of need. It is important to define and elucidate the problem as a whole and further define all the technical and unusual terms employed in the statement.

It is a statement of the limits or scope of the investigation. It will determine the boundaries of the project in hand.

Justification of the Problem: This step would prevent wastage of research efforts on un-important or insignificant problems. The researcher would assess to what extent the solution of the problem would contribute for the furtherance of human knowledge.

Common Errors

(i) Choosing broad area of study

(ii) Impossible for investigation

(iii) Too narrow/small and insignificant topic
(iv) Unscientific, emotional or biased nature
(v) Lack of precision in the instruments.

Steps in Defining Research Problem

The following steps are followed in defining the research problem:

(1) **Statement of problem in a general way:** The problem should be stated in a broad general way, keeping in view either some practical concern or some scientific or intellectual interest.

(2) **Understanding the nature of the problem:** It should be discussed with those who first raised it in order to find out how the problem originally came about and with objectives in view.

(3) **Surveying the available literature:** The problem at hand must necessarily be surveyed and examined before defining a research problem. The researcher must be well conversant with relevant theories in the field reports, records etc.

(4) **Developing the ides through discussions:** The researcher must discuss his problem with his colleagues and others who have enough experience in the same area or in working on similar problems.

(5) **Rephrasing the research problem:** Finally, the researcher must sit to rephrase the research problem into a working proposition. Through rephrasing, the researcher puts the research problem in as specific terms as possible so that it may become operationally viable and may help in the development of working hypothesis.

R.L. Ackoff visualizes the following components of a research problem, namely:

- Research-consumer
- Research-consumer's objectives
- Alternative means to meet the objective
- Doubt in regard to selection of alternatives.

Criteria of a Good Problem Statement

A good problem selected by the researcher should conform to the following criteria: Firstly, the problem should express a relation between two or more variables. It asks question like – is A related to B? How is A related to B?

Secondly, the problem should be related clearly and unambiguously in question form. Instead of saying – "The problem is ....." "The purpose of the study is...." "asks a question". Questions have virtue of posing problems directly. A problem is then an interrogative sentence or statement that asks:

What relation exists between two or more variables? The answer to the question is what is being sought in the research? For example, do teacher comments cause improvement in student performance? What are the effects on pupil performance of different types of incentives?

Thirdly, the problem should be such as to imply possibilities of empirical testing. This means not only that an actual relation is stated, but also that the variables of the relation can somehow be measured.

Normally, the researchers select any particular problem based upon several factors. The following factors may direct the scholar to prefer one topic over the others:

1. To satisfy a personal interest or curiosity,
2. To furnish a basis for conforming some earlier study or a basis for some future study,
3. To meet a social need, or
4. To serve utilization purpose like personal ambition.

The criteria for the selection of a problem may be: interest of the researcher amenability of the problem for research and feasibility of the problem from the point of view of resources. Goods and Half give the following criteria for the selection of a problem:

1. The researcher's interest, intellectual curiosity and drive,
2. Practicability,
3. The urgency of the problem,
4. Anticipating or expected outcomes. Their importance for the field represented and implementation, and
5. Resources, training and personal qualifications of the personnel; availability of special equipment, data, methods, time and sponsorship and administrator's cooperation. A number of criteria in the form of conditions might be listed for guidance in the selection of a topic: (1) Novelty, (2) Interesting, (3) Importance, (4) Feasibility or Amenability, (5) Availability of data, (6) Availability of cooperation, (7) Availability of guidance, (8) Availability of other facilities, (9) Immediate application, (10) Aim of research, (11) Level of research, (12) Experience and creativity, and (13) Courage and confidence.

Similarly Cocharan and Cox suggest that the prospective researcher should put the following questions and select the problems for research:

1. Does the field appeal to my interest?
   (a) Is the interest purely intellectual?
   (b) Is the interest present because of reward of pecuniary returns, possibility in advancement in position and increased authority?
2. Will the result be of practical or utilitarian significance?
3. Does the field present gaps in verified knowledge which need to be filled?

4. Does the field require reworking or reaching?
5. Does the field permit extension of inquiry beyond the present limits or verified knowledge?
6. Is the field pivotal or strategic from the stand point of immediate purpose and the result of the proposed investigation is to be fulfilled?

Notwithstanding the different criteria discussed above, the selection of a research problem remains a difficult and trickles aspect of research, particularly to the uninitiated. Apart from the criteria discussed above, study of the literature on the topic and the related topics, and discussions with persons who have direct knowledge and practical experience in the field would immensely help the researcher in the selection of a problem.

Selection of problem, however, raises two important issues, viz. whether the problem should be selected keeping in view its scientific significance and ethical neutrality or its importance from social, political or historical points of view or its implications for human welfare.

Talcott Parsons, for example, advanced the following point of view: "It is not a question of whether we try to live up to our social responsibilities, but of how. If we should put the overwhelming bulk of our resources, especially on trained talent into immediately practical problems, it would do some good – but I have no doubt that it would have to be at the expenses of our greater usefulness to society in future." For, it is only but systematic work on problem where probable scientific significance has priority over any immediate possibility of application that the greatest and most rapid scientific advance can be made. Parsons position states the importance of "scientific" definitions which focus on immediate practical problems.

C. Wright Mills takes the opposite stance in viewing the selection of problems: "–whether he is aware of it or not any one who spends his life in studying society and publishing the result is actually morally and usually, politically as well. The question is whether he forces this condition and makes up his own mind or whether he conceals it from himself and from others and drifts morally. Many, I should say most, social scientists in America today are easily or uneasily liberal. They conform to the prevailing fear of any passionate commitment. This and not "scientific objectivity" is what is really wanted by such men when they complain about making value judgement".

Mill's argument is that social scientists often use scientific objectivity as an excuse for an uncritical acceptance of the framework of society and that as a result they have spend their intellectual force "on the details of some small scale milieu" instead of concentrating on the large problems of society.

Parsons position stresses the importance of allowing latitude for the investigator to define problems in terms of their 'scientific' significance. Mills maintains that those who profess it tend to take the safe road of avoiding a certain class of those scientific problems, the conclusions of which may imply fundamental criticism of social institutions.

It seems that the debate has pointed up a central question. Which strategies for the selection of problems can maximize the advancement of scientific knowledge as well as the solution of important human problems?

The Academic Research Project

The academic research project is usually a requirement in partial fulfillment of the a postgraduate degree programme – M.A., M.B.A., M.Sc., or for an advanced degree programme like M.Phil. Few such studies make a significant contribution to the field of study or refinement of knowledge. But these research studies help the students to develop some research competency. Most of the postgraduate students tend to select narrow practical problems that rarely contribute to theory.

Levels of Research Projects

Levels of the research will depend upon the purposes of research projects. The first research project because of the limitations of time and other factors emphasised on learning process. The subsequent investigations will yield more significant contributions to the knowledge. The first study, thus, serves as an exploratory process.

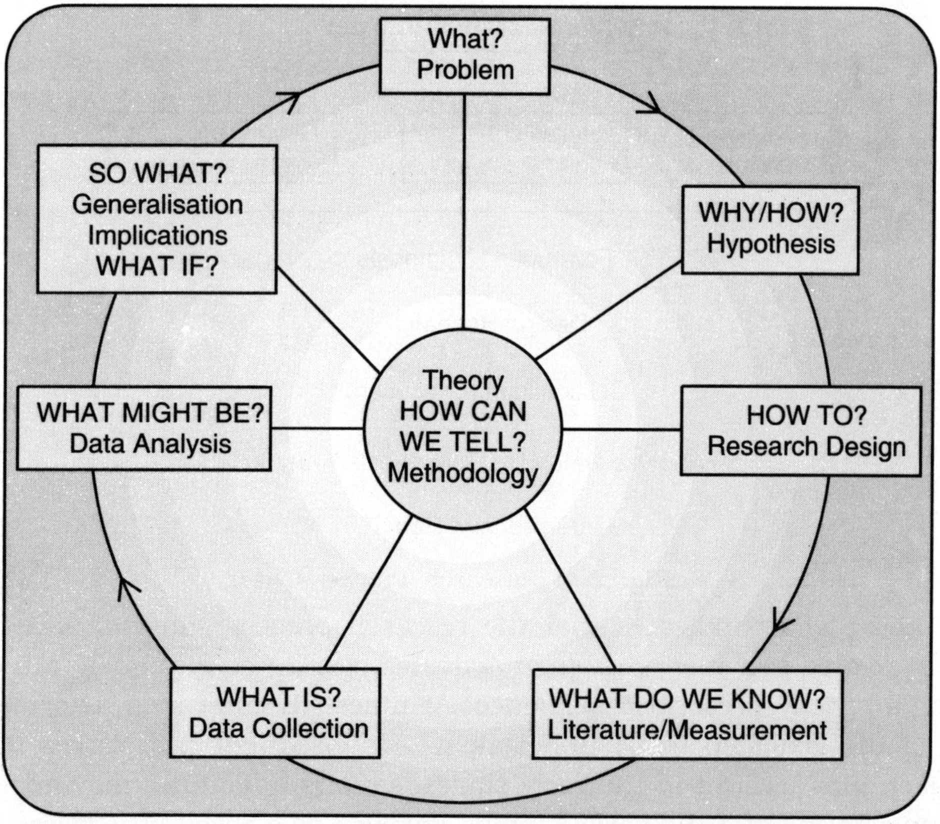

Fig. 2.3: The Research Cycle (*Adapted from Frankfort-Nachmias and Nachmias*).

Some students choose a first problem that can be exploded later into a more comprehensive treatment at the Ph.D. or doctoral level.

There are certain cyclical processes of discovery and analysis. The process of research consists of deciding **why** we want to research, **what** we want to research and **how** we think we are going to do it (the planning phase). Subsequently, we decide **how to** actually do the research and then do it (what data we will collect and how, and then what we will do with these data when we have got them). Finally, we present the results of our efforts. Now, as a result of our research, we think we know something which was not known before, and so are in a position to ask and answer the question: **so what**? (Harvey, n.d.). Frankfort-Nachmias and Nachmias referred to in the above figure has been viewed as old-fashioned and overly empiricist in using the words 'Data Collection' and 'Data Analysis' but data do not have to be positivist or quantitative to be analyzed.

RESEARCH PROCESS

Research process consists of series of action or steps necessary to effectively carry out research and the desired sequencing of these steps.

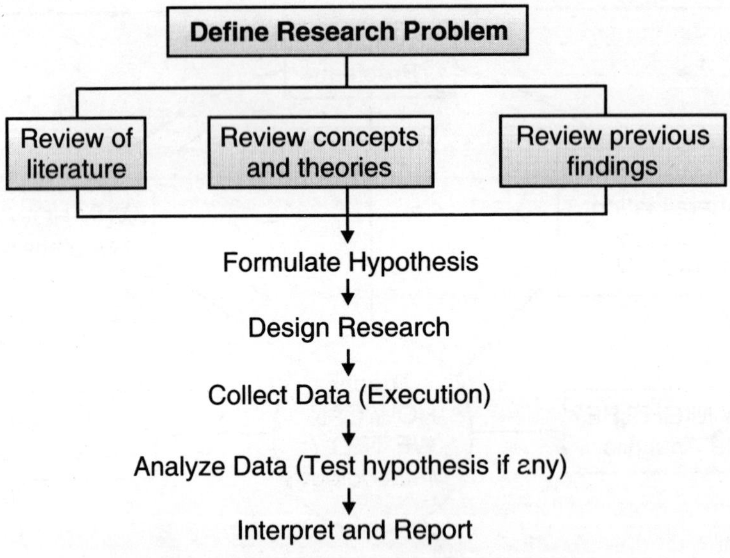

Fig. 2.4: Research Process-Chart.

The above chart indicates that the research process consists of a number of closely related activities. But such activities overlap continuously rather than following a strictly prescribed sequence. At times, the first step determines the nature of the last step to be undertaken. If subsequent procedures have not been taken into account in the early stages, serious difficulties may arise which may even prevent that the various steps involved in a research process are not mutually exclusive; nor are they separate and distinct.

Step 1: Formulating the Research Problem

There are two types of research problems, viz., those which relate to state or nature and those which relates to relationships between variables. At the very outset the researcher must single out the problem he wants to study, i.e., he must decide the general area of interest on aspect of a subject matter that he would like to inquire into. Initially the problem may be stated in a broad general way and then the ambiguities, if any, relating to the problem be resolved. Then, the feasibility of a particular solution has to be considered before a working formulation of the problem can be set up. The formulation of a general topic into a specific research problem constitutes the first step in scientific enquiry. Essentially two steps are involved in formulating the research problem, viz. understanding the problem thoroughly and rephrasing the same into meaningful terms from an analytical point of view.

Step 2: Extensive Literature Survey

The researcher should undertake extensive literature survey connected with the problem. The earlier studies, if any which are similar to the study in hand should be carefully studied. A good library will be a great help to the researcher at this stage.

Step 3: Development of Working Hypothesis

After extensive literature survey, researcher should state in clear terms the working hypothesis or hypotheses. Working hypothesis is a tentative assumption made in order to draw out and test its logical or empirical consequences. As such the manner in which research hypotheses are developed is particularly important since they provide the focal point for research. They also affect the manner in which tests must be conducted in the analysis of data and indirectly the quality of data which is required for the analysis. Hypothesis should be very specific and limited to the piece of research in hand because it has to be tested delimiting the area of research and to keep him on the more important facets of the problem. It also indicates the type of data required and the type of methods of data analysis to be used.

Step 4: Preparing the Research Design

The research problems having been formulated in clear cut terms, the researcher will be required to prepare a research design, i.e., he will have to state the conceptual structure within which research would be as efficient as possible yielding maximal information. In other words, the function of research deigns is to provide for the collection of relevant evidence with minimal expenditure of effort time and money. But how all these can be achieved depends mainly on the research purpose. The research purposes may be grouped into four categories, viz., (i) Exploration, (ii) Description, (iii) Diagnosis, and (iv) Minimizes bias and maximizes the reliability of the data collected and analyzed.

Step 5: Determining the Sample Design

All the items under consideration in any field of inquiry constitutes a 'universe' or 'population'. A complete enumeration of all the items in the population is known as a census inquiry. Besides, this type of inquiry involves a great deal of time, money, and energy. Census inquiry is not possible under many circumstances. For instance, blood testing is done only on sample basis. Hence, quite often we select only a few items from the universe for our study purpose. The items so selected constitute what is technically called a sample or what is popularly known as the sample design.

Step 6: Collecting the Data

In dealing with any real life problem it is often found that data at hand are inadequate, and hence, it becomes necessary to collect data which are appropriate. There are several ways of collecting the appropriate data which differ considerably in context of money costs, time and other resource at the disposal of the researcher. Dr. A.L. Bowley very aptly remarked that in the collection of statistical data, commonsense is the chief requisite and experience the chief teacher.

Step 7: Execution of the Project

Execution of the project is a very important step in the research process. If the execution of the project proceeds on correct lines the data to be collected would be adequate and dependable. The researcher should see that the project is executed in a systematic manner and in time. If the survey is to be conducted by means of a structured questionnaire data can be readily machine-processed. In such a situation, questions as well as the possible answers may be coded. If the data are to be collected through interviewers, arrangements should be made for proper selection and training of the interviewers. They must do their assigned job sincerely and efficiently.

Step 8: Analysis of Data

The analysis of data requires a number of closely related operations such as establishment of categories, the application of these categories to raw data through coding, tabulation and then statistical inferences. Researcher should classify the raw data into some purposeful and usable categories. Coding operation is usually done at this stage through which the categories of data are transformed into symbols that may be tabulated and counted. Editing is the procedure that improves the quality of the data for coding. With coding, the stage is ready for tabulation. Tabulation is a part of the technical procedure wherein the classified data are put in the form of tables. The mechanical devices can be made use of at this juncture. A great deal of data, specially in large inquiries, is tabulated by computers. Computers not only save time but also make it possible to study large number of variables affecting a problem simultaneously.

Step 9: Hypothesis-testing

After analyzing the data as stated earlier, the researcher is in a position to test the hypothesis, if any, he had formulated earlier. Do the facts support the hypothesis or they happen to be contrary? This is the usual question which should be answered while testing hypotheses. Various tests, such as chi-square, t-test, F-test have been developed by statisticians for the purpose. The hypotheses may be tested through the use of one or more of such tests, depending upon the nature and object of research inquiry. Hypothesis-testing will result in either accepting the hypothesis or in rejecting it. If the researcher had no hypotheses to start with, generalization established on the basis of data may be stated as hypotheses which is to be tested by subsequent researcher in times to come.

Step 10: Generalizations and Interpretation

If a hypothesis is tested and upheld several times, it may be possible for the researcher to arrive at generalization, i.e., to build a theory. As a matter of fact the real value of research lies in its ability to arrive at certain generalizations. If the researcher had no hypothesis to start with, he might seek to explain his findings on the basis of some theory. It is known as interpretation. The process of interpretation may quite often trigger off new questions which in turn may lead to further researches.

Step 11. Preparation of the Report or the Thesis

Finally, the researcher has to prepare the report of what has been done by him. Writing of report must be done with great care. Finally, at the end of the report, appendices should be enlisted in respect of all technical data. Bibliography should also be given. Index should also be given specially in a published research report.

In short, the process of research consists of deciding **why** we want to research, **what** we want to research, and how we think we are going to do it (the planning phase). Subsequently, we decide how to actually do the research and then do it (which data we will collect and now, and then what we will do with these data when we have got them). Finally, we present the results of our efforts. Now, as a result of our research, we think we know something which was not known before, and so are in a position to ask and answer the question: **so what**? (Harvey, n.d.).

The approach of Frankfort-Nachmias and Nachmias has been viewed as old-fashioned and overly empiricist in using the words "Data Collection" and "Data Analysis" but data do not have to be positivist or quantitative to be analyzed.

Policy Research: It is basically the research with policy implications. Researches which are conducted for the specific purpose of application or with policy implications may be treated as policy researches. The results of such studies are used as indices for policy formulations and implementation. Many management researches are policy researches. Other types of researches are presented in the next chapter.

Characteristic Features of Scientific Research

(i) **Purposiveness.**

(ii) **Rigor** (carefulness, scrupulousness and the degree of exactness).

(iii) **Replicability:** (The results of the test hypothesis should be supported again and again when the same type of research is repeated in other similar circumstances).

(iv) **Precision and confidence.**

(v) **Parsimony** (simply and economical).

(vi) **Testability.**

(vii) **Objectivity.**

(viii) **Generalizability.**

CHAPTER 3

Types of Research

TYPES OF RESEARCH

1. Historical research (Method)
2. Basic or fundamental or pure or theoretical research vs. Applied and developmental research
3. Quantitative vs. qualitative research
4. Conceptual vs. empirical research
5. Descriptive vs. analytical research
6. Laboratory research
7. Clinical or diagnostic research
8. Exploratory research
9. Survey method
10. Case study method
11. Experimental method
12. Informative systems research
13. Action research
14. Business game
15. Evaluation research.

IMPORTANCE OF KNOWING THE RESEARCH METHODOLOGY

The study of Research Methodology gives the student the necessary training in gathering materials and arranging or card indexing them, participation in the field work when required, and also training in techniques for the collection of data appropriate to particular problems, in the use of Statistics, questionnaires and controlled experimentation and in recording evidence, sorting it out and interpreting it.

(a) **It gives good training to the research worker:** The knowledge of methodology provides good training to the new research worker and enables him to do better research. It helps him to develop disciplined thinking to observe the field objectively.

(b) **Knowledge of research methodology inculcates the ability to evaluate the results:** The researcher will be able to evaluate the results with confidence. The knowledge of Research methodology is helpful in various fields such as Government or business administration, etc.

(c) **Knowledge of research methodology leads to intelligent decisions:** When one comes to know how the research is done, then he may have the satisfaction of acquiring a new intellectual tool which can become a way of looking at the world and of judging every day experience. The knowledge of research methodology provides tools to look at things in life objectively.

(d) **It leads to take rational decisions:** When we are able to judge the adequacy of the methods by which the results have been obtained, then we are able to use them intelligently and take rational decisions.

Research forms the basis of planning, policy making, development of corporate strategy and so on. It is also widely used in the framing of Government policies and social stratification, whether they are social organizations, the Government Educational institutions, or corporate bodies, they all conduct or rely on research findings one time or the other. As students of the course, it is befitting that you gain some insight into the field of research and research methodology. This basic knowledge of research is necessary of everybody more so for managers. In this subject on Research Methodology, an attempt has been made to outline the various types of research, framing of hypothesis, sources and tools of data collection and reporting.

Basis for All Government Policies in Our Economic System

Government Budget is being prepared taking into account the needs and desire of the people. The Government must also consider the position of its revenues. The Government has to take a correct decision. Decision making may not be a part of research, but research certainly facilities the decisions of the policy-maker. Research is considered necessary with regard to the allocation of nation's resources. The Government would also like to collect information regarding the economic and social structure of the nation. Collecting such statistical information involves a variety of research problems.

SOLVING OPERATIONAL AND PLANNING PROBLEMS OF BUSINESS AND INDUSTRY

For Business decisions, Marketing Research and Operations Research are conducted, Market Research is the investigation of the structure and development of a market for the purpose of formulating efficient policies for Purchasing, Production and Sales. Operations research refers to the application of mathematical, logical and analytical techniques to the solution of business problems of cost minimization or of profit maximization. Research with regard to demand and market factors has great utility in business. Market analysis has become an integral tool of business policy. Now-a-days, Business budgeting results in a projected profit and loss account, based mainly on sales estimates which in turn depends on business research.

HISTORICAL METHOD/RESEARCH

In 1961 Carr wrote the book "What is History?". E.H. Carr's 14-volume history of the creation and early years of the Soviet Union directly influenced ones conception of how to undertake historical research. Hayden White (1973) has suggested that writing 'history' and writing 'fiction' have much in common. The former appears to require 'finding' rather 'inventing' facts. 'Fiction' refers to something that are invented or imagined. It may suggest the ways and means to avoid a difficult situation.

History has all along been a great source of inspiration for researchers. In fact, there is considerable research which can be done only with the help and assistance of historical data and as such historical method for the study of social research occupies a very significant place. According to Walter R. Borg, 'Historical Research is the systematic and synthesis–objective location, evaluation synthesis of evidence in order to establish facts and draw conclusions concerning past events.' To quote P.V. Young, 'The past, if it can be located, contains the key to the present, though today is different from yesterday, it was shaped by yesterday, Today and yesterday will probably influence tomorrow'. Historical method is specially useful and important for social scientists because it is with their help that they understand the social change on the one hand and growth of social institutions and organizations on the other. It has been very appropriately said that past contains key to the present. Any research which makes use of observations based on past events is known as research in historical approach.

In the past, history was considered nothing else but recording of past events. Then history did not contain anything else but only deeds and misdeeds of the ruling monarchs. Usually, however, whereas the deeds were exaggerated, misdeeds were minimized with the result that even the events narrated were undependable and needed careful scrutiny before acceptance. But now the approach has changed and history is being written with different objective. The history is not the mere narration of past events and deeds and misdeeds of the monarch but these include information about social institutions, social organizations, masses, their economic, political, social and cultural conditions. The history records, social systems and phenomenon. In history, the role of social events in the life of the people began to be depicted. In the present history a prominent place is being assigned to various classes of people. In the present history, a prominent place is being assigned to class struggle which is going between different classes, e.g., the capitalists, agriculturists and workers etc. Our present historians have now come to realize that the events in society can take place without social background and that every event should be studied with that background. The new approach has, thus, brought society very near. Social research increasingly realized that social forces play a big role in socio economic and political life of the country. It is, therefore, being accepted that history is very useful source of social research. It provides material for the study of very social institution and that social change and progress can best be appreciated with the help of history.

Sources of Historical Data

(i) Autobiographies
(ii) Memories, personal letters and accounts
(iii) Diaries and confessions
(iv) Books and magazines
(v) Scared archives
(vi) Assessable documents, papers and literature
(vii) Diplomatic agreements
(viii) Personal sources of authentic observers and witnesses
(ix) Cultural and analytical history material
(x) Artistic materials, historical paintings, portraits, charts, maps
(xi) Statistical materials etc.

Steps in Historical Methods

In so far as historical method for the study of social problem is concerned, there are certain steps involved in that, before a social investigator can usefully use and employ that method. First step is selection of problem. All problems cannot be solved with the help of historical method. Of course, it will have to be seen that only such problems are picked up which need scanning of historical records. No current problem can usefully and proposefully be studied with the help of this method. Needless to say that before picking up the problem one has to see that it is social utility and that it is not too expensive.

After the problem has been selected for research and it has been decided that the matter will be collected with the help of historical records, then the question of collecting data will arise. In so far as data collection is concerned, it can be collected with the help of either primary or secondary sources. Primary sources include autobiographies, documents, diaries of the people written by them, whereas secondary sources include such publicized works etc., which do not record the event by the eye witnesses but were recorded at some later date. In such cases, information is collected by the people from different sources and then recorded in a way which is liked by the person who has collected information. Obviously, primary sources of data collection are more important than the secondary sources.

After the data has been collected, problem of generalization and analysis comes. A this stage what the researcher will have to see is that the date has been fully collected and that nothing has been left out. If any source of material has been left out that will create the problem of tilting the findings either on this side. It can be either exaggeration of facts from one side or that of understanding on the other.

Sources of Historical Data

From which source can historical data be selected is another problem which needs consideration. These sources are documents, materials of cultural history and personal sources of authentic observers and witnesses. In what way is each source to be tackled will depend on the student on the one hand and nature or problem on the other.

Direct use of documents will prove more useful and advantageous when:

(i) Events which these documents have not yet been analyzed by the historians.

(ii) When these events have not been incorporated into writings.

(iii) When the basic idea is to verify certain events directly.

(iv) When certain aspects of life in which investigators are interested have not been embodied in the later writings of analytical historians.

(v) When there is a missing link in knowledge and that need be connected as that whole event becomes complete about a social situation.

(vi) When there is incomplete chronology of events.

(vii) When a controversial point needs to be settled.

PRECAUTIONS IN THE USE OF HISTORICAL DATA

Historical data will have to be used with great care and consideration, otherwise the results to the desired extent might not be achieved. First precaution is that the investigator should not use only such data which is easily available and leave what he considers will be difficult to lay hand on. Then another precaution which should take is that the investigator should not over generalize the findings of his study. In other words, he should give proper importance to specific and specialized events, so that the whole problem is studied in right perspective and manner. Then another care which the investigator will have to distinguish is that in what sense the terms was used in the past and in what sense it is being used in the present. Obviously, if the same term is being used in different senses that would convey different meaning and that will have to be appreciated. In case this basic difference is not appreciated, whole study will become defective.

NECESSARY CONDITIONS FOR HISTORICAL RESEARCH

(i) Selection of topic for research

(ii) Familiarity with the topic and its objectives

(iii) Knowledge of study field

(iv) Availability of necessary facilities

(v) Selection and rejection of the material

(vi) Social insight

(vii) Historical orientation

(viii) Knowledge of related social sciences.

Advantages of Historical Methods

(i) Historical method fills in a big gap of making the research possible and also meaningful on the problems that would otherwise have remained unexplored.

(ii) It has an advantage to offer the past data under the then prevailing conditions and afford an opportunity to the researcher to view these observations in the past setting.

(iii) Historical records provide very useful information that goes a long way towards the solution of a research problem.

Limitations of Historical Method

Though historical method has its own importance in the study of social research, yet this method has its own limitations as well. Real good results can only be obtained with help of this method provided these limitations are removed to the extent possible. Some of the important limitations are dearth of reliable data, availability of record keeping, dispersal of documents, problems of frame of conditioning phenomenon, no test or verification, problem of calculation and measurement of data and the problem of bias. To sum up:

(i) A serious shortcoming is that any past situation cannot be matched to an existing situation.

(ii) Researchers tend to over-generalize their results.

(iii) Sometimes researcher adopts a subjective interpretation in order to validate his hypothesis. The loss of objectivity in such cases can lead to considerable inaccuracies in research findings.

(iv) Limitations may also arise in the writing of history itself because of personal biases. Moreover, not all happenings in time and space can be known at the time of writing.

Contribution of Historical Method of Social Science

Historical method has come to stay as one of the important methods for the study of social sciences and historians in this way have contributed a lot in so far as study of social problems is concerned. It is with the help of this data that comparative data can be collected for verifying the hypothesis once developed. History provides diversified information to prove the weakness of strength of every theory. It is that historical data which provides many useful clues for understanding many unknown social problem. With the help of this method, realistic bias can be provided for measuring factors in the formulation of social theory. It is with the help of this method that knowledge or circumstances and conditions in which an experiment took place can be obtained. In other words, it is with the help of this method that we come to know how a particular idea was conceived and if the experiment failed, what were its important causes.

Historical Method in Modern Times

In our modern times historical method is being more and more increasingly used. It is now being realized that even social institutions, organizations and systems have historical background and in case that background is not properly studied, whole study will be incomplete. Today, such important institutions are those of family, divorce, caste system etc. being studied more seriously with the help of historical method.

Of course, there are thinkers in social sciences who believe that his method should not be extensively used in social science because it is undependable and unreliable. Much of the data is more imaginative and subjective rather than realistic and objective. They also feel that the myth, fiction and reality in historical documents are so much fixed up that it is different to separate the two.

History is providing a lot of material for the study of social problems. In a right way, it is giving a useful information about growth as well as fall of many social, economic and political institutions. In other words, history provides information and also gives a warning to our social researchers, so that they do not go astray and keep a track of the work undertaken by them.

BASIC OR FUNDAMENTAL OR PURE OR THEORETICAL RESEARCH VS. APPLIED AND DEVELOPMENTAL RESEARCH

By basic research, we mean the investigation of problems in order to further and develop existing knowledge. It is concerned with the generalization and with the formulation of a theory. Gathering knowledge for knowledge sake is termed basic research.

The distinction between pure (or basic or fundamental) and applied research needs some elaboration. Basic research helps to extend the frontiers of knowledge. It helps evolving of new theories, brings theories nearer to world of real and modifies existing theories in relation to changes in institution and ideologies. As the perfectly competitive market model in modern economics was found to be unrealistic, Chamberlin and Mrs. Joan Robinson evolved their theories of monopolistic and imperfect competition. Galbraith's New Industrial State expounds the rule of the technocrats and the erosion of the profit maximization principle. Other examples are Cobb-Douglas Production Function, Minhas' C.E.S. production function, linear programming evolved by Chenery, Kantoroitch, Ragnar Frisch and Jan Tin Bergen. The basic research is light-yielding and the researcher is a tool-maker. Classical economic theories are based on the postulate of harmony between classes; Marxian philosophy stresses conflict and class-war which has led to formulation of distinct theories. Both the capitalistic and socialistic theories are not adequate to a proper understanding of the mixed economies. The evolution of joint partnership between the public and private sectors, commended by Alvin Hansen for the U.S.A. needs formulation of fresh theories. With every change in the structure of the economy and in the economic philosophy, we need few more theories.

The so-called Third World of developing economies are primarily low-income countries, with appalling poverty, enormous unutilized manpower, meagre capital and insatiable demand for consumption goods. The theories, applicable to developed economies, including Keynesian theory of underemployment equilibrium, do not appear to be relevant to Under Development Countries (UDC). The dichotomy of their economies into isles of industrialized sector and seas of subsistence sector calls for a new set of theories to gain a correct understanding of their working and behaviour. Theories of economic growth evolved in and applicable to developed countries do not solve the problem of UDC. To argue that scientific theories should be universal in their application in all climat and at all times is to turn one's eyes away from the realities. Social and economic laws are not universal like the laws of natural sciences, because of differences between and changes in institution, ideologies, attitudes, customs and prejudices of the various groups of people. Further, in the poor developing economies, free enterprise is curbed by price control and factor allocation, widening public sector, factor immobility, exchange control, import and export quotas. Nor is there so much of absolute state control and central planning as in communistic countries to warrant the applicability of socialistic theories? Hence, there is a real need for theories suitable to the UDC. That the flame of pure research should be kept ever burning all the time, in every country ever brighter, needs no further argument.

Applied research is problem-oriented. It helps the choice of policies, determination of priorities, formulation and appraisal of projects. During the phase of economic development in UDC, several problems crop up, calling for investigation and solutions. In the developed countries too, the constant flux and dynamism of the economies throw up several problems, e.g., stagnation and the array of problems exposed in Galbraith's 'Affluent Society', Boulding's description of the economist as an 'information animal' and of the politician as a decision-making animal underlines the duties of investigation on the part of the economist, to gain knowledge and feed the decision makers. The problems are a legion, those of the public and private sectors, regional and national projects, evaluation and projection, inflation and unemployment, effects of tax-cuts and budget-deficits, changes in wages, bonuses and D.A., attitudes of consumers and producers, demand forecast to guide the policy of demand management, benefit-cost evaluation, man-power studies, family planning-knowledge, application and practice, green revolution, mobilization of rural savings, sick textile mills, progress of industrial estates, wastages and cost of education, housing rural employment, assessing welfare of Harijans, tribal people, foreign loan, aid, investment and collaboration, public and private sectors collaboration, etc.

Applied economic researcher is mainly a tool-user and his research is fruit-yielding. However, no rigid separation between basic and applied research exists. Not infrequently applied research spotlights the week points in the existing theories and indicates the lines on which pure research should be initiated. There is still a lingering suspicion that basic is superior to applied research. The latter, being problem-oriented and often of trouble shooting type, is engrossed in present day transient problems. Applied researchers are inclined to feel infra dig. Basic research calls for actions to remove hazards and to enjoy the delight of exploration. It may end just like oil or diamond prospecting; one may either gloriously succeed in discovering the mine or after laborious, prolonged and vain search end in dismal failure. Applied research is indeed the art, used by the practitioners of science. What is the use of a science if its tools are not applied to solve the real work problems?

Max Millikan once, of course, lamented on the level of pure theory, India has still not made frontier contribution to the analysis of growth – economic growth which one might hope from a country as fully embarked as she has experiment of consciously promoting such growth. This is an adverse criticism on us. Marshall's advice to Schumpeter applies comforting function to hurt the conscience of the Indian researchers. Diminishing returns have already set in there. The world is waiting for a thousand important applications' in research development.

1. **Quantitative Vs. Qualitative Research:** The former is based on the measurement of quantity and the latter is concerned with phenomena relating to or involving kind/quality. Motivation research is an important type of quality research. The partnership between quantitative, demographic, statistical evidence and qualitative exemplars or paradigms perhaps brings us nearer to grail of Social Care Model (Ideology).

Types of Qualitative Research: (i) Ethnography, Case study research, Phenomenological research, and Grounded theory.

Ethnography: The word ethnography is derived from the Greek words ethos ('tribe') and graphos ('something that is written'). Literally, then, ethnography is the science of writing about tribes or, to use contemporary language, writing about cultural groups. Ethnographic researchers hope to provide rich narratives or descriptions of the communities or cultures under invstigation (Miles & Huberman, 1994).

Phenomenological Research: It looks closely at an individual's interpretation of his or her experiences. Phenomenologists attempts to understand the manning of an experience from the perspective of the participants. Wanting to understand the human experience and how experiences are interpreted differently by different people would certainly be an appropriate reason to conduct a phenomenological study.

Grounded Theory Research uses the inductive approach and collects data using multiple techniques over a long period of time. The data collected are continually reviewed to build a theory that is 'grounded' in the data. This method is based on the work of Glaser and Strauss (1967), who are generally responsible for the introduction of this approach. These kinds of studies do not result in a theory such as Piaget's theory of cognitive development or Freud's psychosexual theory. Grounded theories are practical theories that are designed to be used in the context of the field studied, as well as in other similar settings. Grounded theorists differ from other qualitative researchers in that they hope that their findings can be generalized to other settings. Grounded-theory researchers have refined the process of analyzing qualitative data and use the term **'constant comparison'** to describe this sophisticated method of data analysis.

2. **Conceptual Vs. Empirical Research:** The former is related to some abstract ideas or theory and is used by philosophers and thinkers to develop new concepts or to interpret the existing ones. The latter is data-based research coming up with conclusions which are capable of being verified by observation or experiment.

3. **Descriptive (Ex-post facto) Vs. Analytical/library/Desk Research (method) or Non-Experimental, or Correlational Research:** A descriptive research describer interprets facts as they are, the conditions that exist, the relationship between two events, opinions that are held the processes, that are going on effects, that are evident, and the trends that are developing. Descriptive research involves events that have already taken place and may be related to present conditions and also preliminary what is happening now. Hence, they are called ex-post fact, i.e., fact after it has happened. For example, there was an evaluation of voting behaviour of people in India by different research groups.

In descriptive research the investigator or researcher does not manipulate events. This methods is widely used in behavioural science, because there are many human behaviours which can not be manipulated, and it is also unethical. For example, to study the effect of deprivation of food, a researcher should not deprive children from eating when they are hungry, to understand its effect on lungs. Thus, in studying such relationship, the researcher has to use descriptive methods where human behaviour can be systematically analyzed and examined in natural settings.

However, descriptive studies also have the criteria of science namely, (a) disciplined enquiry, (b) expertise in the field, (c) objectivity, and (d) careful execution.

Descriptive research describes the state of affairs as it exists at present. It describes what is – Economic Survey of Chennai City, Bench-mark survey etc. It includes surveys and fact-finding enquiries of different kinds. Here, the researcher has no control over the variables.

Example for this type of research: Frequency of shopping, preferences of people or similar data. Ex-post facto research is an empirical research and the researcher does not have any control over independent variables. The ex-post facto research may be carried out on a limited scale or on a very large scale depending upon what techniques of research are available with the researcher.

Expost-fact studies or descriptive research methods trend to include attempts by research to discover causes even when they cannot control variables.

One of the serious dangers of these studies is post-hocus-pocus-fallacy, that is, the conclusion that two factors go together one must become the cause and the other must be effect.

The limitations of descriptive research are as follows:

(a) The independent variable cannot be manipulated. (For example, people's preferences for particular brand of the product cannot be manipulated.)

(b) Subjects cannot be randomly assigned to different conditions. (For example, in a cross-section of sample the subjects cannot be classified and grouped.)

(c) Researcher cannot establish cause and effect relation between variables instead they prefer to observe that when variable A appears, variable B is inconsistently associated. Sometimes the causes are often multiple rather than single.

Descriptive studies aim at portraying accurately the characteristics of a particular group or situation. One may undertake a descriptive study about the works in a factory their age distribution, their community wise distribution, their educational level, the state of their physical health and so on and so forth. Also one may study the conditions of work in a factory, Health, safety and welfare. A descriptive study may be concerned with the attitude of views (of people) towards anything, e.g., attitudes towards presidential form of Government, rights to strike, capital punishments, prohibiting college autonomy, widows' marriage etc., the design in such studies must be rigid and not flexible and must involve the following steps:

(a) Formulating the objectives of the study.

(b) Defining the population and selecting a sample.

(c) Designing the methods of data collection.

(d) Processing and analyzing the data.

(e) Reporting the findings.

Analytical research (Library or desk research): In analytical research, the researcher uses facts or data already available and analyzes them to make a critical evaluation of the material. The social science researcher uses the library perusing the secondary data as a physical – scientist – researcher would digest the reports on the early experiments.

4. **Laboratory Research:** The emphasis is to control certain variables in such a way to observe the relationship between two or three other variables.

5. **Clinical or Diagnostic Research:** It follows case study methods or in-depth approaches to reach the basic causal relationship. This type of research takes only a few samples and studies the phenomena in-depth and observes the effects.

6. **Exploratory Research (Exploratory method):** The exploratory method, according to Katz, 'represented the earlier stage of science.' This significance observation implies that all sciences must have at the beginning had an approach which was purely exploratory. Even as we approach a doctor with an ailment he starts with all sorts of questions, to begin with. From the point of view of the doctor, he is systematically exploring the complaints and is striving to categorize our symptoms. On the basis of this exploration he will arrive at a conclusion, at least tentatively, about the disease. Only then will he, if necessary, call for a pathological report. All these steps, starting with the exploratory questions will help him to arrive at a correct diagnosis. This example will, while making the meaning of exploration clear, also point out the inevitability and universability of the exploratory approach, which cuts across the barrier of the natural and social sciences. At this stage one may be tempted to conclude that the moment one envisages his study as exploratory, the investigator has absolute freedom for random and aimless activity. The social scientist has freedom to follow interesting leads and to utilize his own ingenuity in obtaining information. Yet, the social scientist should exercise judicious temperance in this approach. Man's knowledge of the social sciences has progressed to a degree where social scientists do have knowledge of "The types of things to look for in most social situations" (Katz, 1953).

With this it should be clear that the exploratory study is systematic. Scientific, and at times the only way through which a social scientist can check whether an idea, that sounds promising to him has much appeal, if at all, in reality or not. In fact, exploratory studies can provide ideas, hypotheses or suggestions that might never occur to a social scientist sitting in an office and meditating over the problem.

The major advantage of the exploratory method lies in its ability to generate many ideas that could be further explored in more controlled conditions, apart from overcoming the most difficult portion of an inquiry, which is its initiation. It also safeguards social scientists from the possible future embarrassment of having spent a tremendous amount of energy and time and of having squandered the scarce resources. What is more, it will also in the long run save him from rancour for having arrived at results which at best could be described as sterile. Katz goes to the extend of suggesting that even an exploratory study should be so designed as to provide as definite information as possible for a set of research objectives. "In order to attain research objectives" the exploratory method, as suggested by Selltiz et al., should adopt the following steps:

1. **Review of related social science and other pertinent literature:** One of the simplest ways of economizing effort in an inquiry is to review the work already done by others. The information, thus, gathered will serve as leads for further investigation. Careful review of the availability material will be helpful in deriving a workable hypotheses with precise meaning. They also suggest important variables for a social scientist.

2. **Survey of people who had practical experience with the problem to be studied:** Persons by virtue of the nature of their jobs are in a position to throw light on the subject matter of interest to the investigator. Such knowledgeable and experienced persons should not be ignored. "Such specialists acquire, in the routine of their work, a reservoir of experience that could be of tremendous value in helping the social scientist to become aware of the important influences operating in any situation he may be called upon to study". An investigator at the same time should remember that in an experience survey it is a waste of time and effort to interview people who have little competence or little relevant experience or who lack ability to communicate their experiences.

3. **The analysis of insight-stimulating examples:** Social scientists working in an area which is yet to be explored, which incidentally is the usual experience of an innovative social scientist, have found intensive study of the selected samples to be particularly fruitful method of stimulating insight. For

example, remarkable theoretical insights of Sigmund Freud were the result of stimulation provided by his intensive studies of patients. Profound changes in our conception of the relationship between man and society have been brought about largely by intensive anthropological studies of primitive cultures. It will be beneficial for the evoking of insight if the attitude of the investigator is one of alert receptivity, of seeking rather than testing. An investigator should remember that this inquiry is constantly in the process of reformulation and redirection as new information is obtained. Lastly, this approach is characterized by its reliance on integrative powers of the investigator, on his ability to draw together many diverse bits of information into a unified interpretation.

Katz has conceptual exploratory studies at two levels; the first is the discovery of the significant variable in the situation and the second is the discovery of relationship between variables. It is imperative for the investigator to delimit the area to be studied specially at the first level. Exploratory studies which do not set matters, some of which may not be realized by the investigator at the formulative stages. The need for exercising some sort of control in collecting or recording respondent's responses will be imminent sooner rather than later. Hence, it will help if the investigator, at formulative stage, is aware of his need for delimiting the problem to be studied. Katz advises that it is much more effective to take one central set of variables and investigate them as thoroughly as possible. The investigator may save himself disappointment if he does not look for discernment – differences which are perhaps likely to be difficult in exploratory studies. Further, they merely lead to insight or hypotheses, but they do not test or demonstrate them. Careful and controlled studies are needed to test whether the hypotheses that emerge out of studies employing the exploratory method have general acceptability and applicability. While discussing the exploratory study as an entity, it is appropriate to consider it as an initial step in a continuous research process. They are undertaken with the explicit purpose of formulating a problem for more precise investigation or for developing hypotheses.

In condition it can be said that no research proposal be aborted for want of methodology, as long as we have the exploratory method. This method is flexible enough to permit the consideration of many different aspects of a phenomenon. This method attempts to see what there is rather than to predict the relationship that will be found. Mostly the results obtained through the exploratory study are to be treated as a sign post for future and further study in the same or similar direction. For this reason they are also known as formulative studies.

The exploratory research (method) according to Katz, 'represents the earlier stage of science'. Katz has conceptualized exploratory studies at two levels: the first is the discovery of the significant variable in the situation and the second is the discovery of relationship between variables. The aim of this type of research is the development of hypothesis rather than their testing.

SURVEY METHOD

The most important method of research very widely used by the researcher in different field is 'survey'. The survey method involves mainly assessment of the status of a phenomenon at a particular time. For example, mock poll survey on voting. It describes without value judgment a situation that prevail; it attempts no explanation of underlying reasons and no recommendation for action. It just deals with prevailing opinion, knowledge or practices of people. Many market surveys try to estimate or assess the people's preferences for various products.

The survey method involves a clearly defined problems and objectives. It requires an expert planning, careful analysis, and interpretation of the data gathered. It needs a great account of logic and skill in reporting the findings. Some popularly known surveys are given below:

Social surveys	–	Peoples awareness about AIDS
	–	Prevalence
Economic surveys	–	How rich is India?
Political surveys	–	Popularity of leaders of various parties as Prime Minister Candidate
Public opinion survey	–	Banning smoking in public places. Wearing helmets for two wheelers

Descriptive research method tries to relate two events or occurrences. Hence, they are called correlational studies. Epidemiological research methods widely use descriptive methods in studying trends and indices of diseases. For example, retrospective studies relate personal histories of smoking with medical and mortality rates.

PILOT SURVEYS

A pilot survey is a small scale replica of the main survey. The pilot survey is a dress rehearsal. The pilot study provides guidance on the following:

(i) The adequacy of the sampling frame to be followed for the survey.

(ii) The pilot study enables the researcher to acquire prior knowledge about the population to be sampled.

(iii) The probable number of refusals and non-contacts can be roughly be estimated from the pilot survey. As a result, a particular data collection method may be chosen in preference to others.

(iv) After examining alternative methods such as observation, questionnaire and interview schedule the suitability of method of collecting the data can be found out from the pilot study.

(v) The pilot study provides scope to find out whether the wording in the questionnaire is simple, clear, unambiguous or free from technical terms.

(vi) The pilot study enables to test the efficiency of the instructions and general briefing of interviews. Sometimes, the instructions may be adequate, but the interviewer may be doing a poor job.

(vii) The pilot study provides training to the interviewers.

(viii) The probable cost and duration of the main survey and its various stages will be known with the help of the pilot study. Pilot survey is valuable if the main survey is too long and too expensive.

The size and design of the pilot survey is a matter of convenience. The sample should be of comparable structure of that of main survey. The sample of the pilot survey must be widespread as the main sample. If two forms of questions are to be compared, each should be tried out. All the technique of processing and analysis of data have to be piloted.

MERITS OF SURVEY METHOD

The survey method has the following merits:

(i) The survey method enables the researcher to come into direct contact with the people whom he wants to study.

(ii) The survey provides scope for the introduction of a new theory. For example, long time poverty was the cause for crime. But the surveys conducted in advanced countries have falsified this theory.

(iii) A survey facilitates the researcher to observe the emotional impact of social situation. The survey method is well suited to study the people with specialized characteristics.

(iv) Surveys are conducted for business purposes. For example, to ascertain the popularity of the products introduced by a business concern.

(v) Survey is meant to provide information regarding practical problems.

(vi) Survey is conducted to investigate some cause and effect relationship.

Demerits of Survey Method

(i) Most of the surveys are conducted on sample basis, and the informant may not become the representative of the universe.

(ii) Survey method lays importance upon current problems. A comprehensive study of the society is not possible.

(iii) Survey method refers to study undertaken for short time. A study involving long term development cannot be undertaken under this method.

(iv) A survey method of research requires a considerable amount of money for printing schedules, for field work training, and supervision, tabulation, and analysis of the data.

(v) Most of the surveys are conducted in a hurry and the reliability and validity of each information is questionable.

(vi) A survey will lead to desired result, if the survey has been perfectly preplanned. But a perfect preplanning is seldom possible.

Steps in Sampling

The process of selecting the sample consists of several steps or procedures. They are as follows:

(1) Defining the survey population or universe.

(2) Specifying the frame of sampling.

(3) Specifying sampling unit.

(4) Specifying method of sampling.

(5) Determining the size of sample.

(6) Deciding the plan for selecting the sampling units.

(7) Actual selection of sample.

Definition of Social Survey

Survey research includes both the census and sample survey, yet it usually means the latter. Survey method is a device for collecting data or factual information of certain desired characteristics or items of a universe or population.

"Social Survey is a fact-finding study dealing chiefly with working class, poverty, and with the nature and problems of community." – *A.F. Wells*

"Survey research is an organized attempt to analyze, interpret and report the present status of social institutions, group or area." – *F.L. Whitney*

"A social survey is a process by which quantitative facts are collected about the social aspect of a community's composition and activities." – *Mark Abrams*

One of the common methods of diagnosing and solving of social problems is that of undertaking surveys. Surveys are of various types and as such these considerably help in solving each type of problem. This method of research has been in vogue to a varying degree since the time past and still continues in use. Social Survey is one of the important methods of social investigation, in so far the scope of investigation is confined to a particular area. It helps in solving problems of a group of community in so far as that is confined to definite geographical limits.

Different definitions have been given to define the scope of this subject. Festinger and Katz are of the opinion that 'Many research problems require systematic collection of data from population through the use of personal interviews or other data gathering devices. These studies are usually called surveys, especially when they are concerned with groups of people'. Mark Abram has defined social survey by saying that 'A social survey is a process by which quantitative facts are collected about the social aspects of a community composition and activities'. Borgardus, E.S. is of the view that "A social survey is the collection of data concerning the living and working conditions, broadly speaking the people in a given community". From these definitions, it will be observed that social survey is a type of survey conducted with a view purpose that general or specific information about society should be collected and complied.

Kinds of Social Survey

(i) **Regular or Ad hoc Survey:** If the survey is repeated for regular intervals to obtain continuous information, it is known as regular survey. Ad hoc surveys are conducted once for all and are non-repetitive. When a body/ individual/organization conducts some survey at regular intervals, say for, e.g., economic survey of the Reserve Bank of India or the census survey by the Registrar General of India, the survey is called regular survey. On other hand, if the survey is conducted with a view to finding out some information required for a particular purpose and the purpose of survey is over, as soon as the object is achieved, the survey is called an ad hoc survey. Obviously, in the case of ad hoc survey the information called for is not of regular nature and that the data collected relates to certain specific matter and is not of any routine nature.

(ii) **Official and Non-official Survey:** A survey can be conducted by the government for finding out certain facts for official as well as philanthropic purposes. Such survey is called official survey. Surveys are also conducted by individuals as well as companies, research organizations with or without the help of the government. Such surveys are called non-official surveys. Needless to say that the surveys conducted by the government are more sound and comprehensive than any other survey, due to availability of more resource and manpower.

(iii) **Preliminary and Final Surveys:** Preliminary survey is the pilot study to get the first hand knowledge of the universe under study. It helps the researcher in preparing schedule or questionnaire and organizing the survey on proper lines. Final surveys are made after the pilot study has been completed.

(iv) **Direct or Indirect Survey:** Surveys have also been classified as direct and indirect surveys, i.e., in former case facts can be quantitatively interpreted whereas in the latter case that is not possible and results are to be concluded out of the available data by some indirect method.

(v) **Personal or Postal Survey:** A personal survey is one in which the surveyor himself is required to move about and collect information personally but on the other hand in the case of postal survey, surveyors get information through post. The methods have their own advantages and disadvantages. Whereas in the case of personal survey the surveyor can also know about the mood, temperament and reliability of information supplied by him. He may not be in a position to get detailed information for want of time. The advantage of detailed and considered opinion being provided is possible only in the postal survey.

(vi) **General or Specific Surveys:** A general survey is conducted for collecting general information of any population, institution or phenomena without any hypothesis, while the specific surveys are conducted for specific problems or for testing the validity of some theory or hypothesis.

(vii) **Census and Sample Survey:** Census is enquiry which involves a complete enumeration or a comprehensive count of all the units of the population. Census survey deals with the investigation of entire population. It is a costly and time-consuming process. Instead of obtaining data from all the units of the universe, sampling survey is conducted. In a sample survey only a small part of the universe which is representative of the whole population is taken and the information is collected.

Objectives of Social Sample Survey

The main objective of the social sample survey is to obtain accurate and reliable information about the universe with minimum of cost, time and energy and to set out the limits of accuracy of such estimates.

Social Surveys are conducted with different objects in view. One such object is that of collecting detailed information about a social problem under investigation. C.A. Moser is of the view that, purpose of many surveys is simply to provide someone an information. That someone may be a government wanting to know how much people spend on food, business concern interested to find out what detergents people are using, a research institute studying the housing of old age pensioners and so on.

Then another objective can be that with the help of social surveys it can be possible to find out problem of social disorganization and social stratification. It becomes then possible to know why society is not progressing in spite of certain legal facilities already provided, e.g., in India a survey could reveal why the scheduled caste and scheduled tribe candidates are not forthcoming for the jobs reserved for them in government departments and public sectors undertaking and so on. Thus a survey is likely to help in finding out explanation of a social phenomenon with some confidence and authenticity. Since the investigator is face to face with respondent, he can get detailed information from the latter and collect his views on the subject under investigation.

Yet another object can be to test hypothesis. Each survey is conducted with some hypothesis. Unless there is a hypothesis, investigator cannot proceed. Whether that hypothesis is right or wrong, sound or unsound is another problem. That needs testing. After the information has been collected with the help of survey then it can be said if the hypothesis has been proved or disproved.

Pre-requisite of a Good Surveyor

A good surveyor cannot start his wok off hand. He must be clear about the nature of his enquiry and also with the type of questionnaire. He must be clear about the fields and areas of study to be covered by him and also the scope and nature of his study. He should be capable enough of delimiting his areas so that the nature of his study does not become too wide. He must also be mentally prepared to utilize both primary as well as secondary sources for his survey. Not only this he should not leave data unutilized and must be prepared to have tabulated analysis of the data which he has collected, by the survey.

Advantages of Social Surveys

Social surveys are really time consuming and also costly and as such those should be conducted with care and conscience. These however, come to stay on account of certain advantages namely:

(a) It is with the help of the surveys that it becomes possible to study a problem thoroughly and deeply, in all aspects. It is only then the causes of the problem can be studied and it can be found out, if the causes are reasonable and that remedies can be used to find a solution to the problem. Since the problems have been properly diagnosed, it is very much hoped that the remedies will prove effective.

(b) Another advantage is that it is very useful for administrators and policy makers. We find that in many states many important legislative measures were taken as a result of findings of social surveys. In fact in many countries working conditions of the poor, backward and the exploited could be remedied only after survey findings were available.

(c) It is with the help of social surveys that the trend of changes as well as disorganization in the society can be found out, as we know that every developing society is witnessing changes. In some cases such changes can be slow, whereas in other cases they can be fast. Similarly in every society certain factors disturb society and causes disorganization in the society. It is only with the help of surveys that such changes, the extent of their gravity and force as well as pressures of public opinions can be found out.

(d) Since in a society survey an investigator himself comes in contact with the people, about whom he wants to know, the facts collected are based on the reality of life. The information collected is dependable and reliable and has great amount of certainty. Accordingly, social surveys are dependable, which is a virtue of social sciences.

(e) No social survey can be conducted and it possible, unless a large number of people are sent to field. According to the chances of objectivity, bias is reduced to the minimum. The bias introduced by one investigator, can hopefully be negatived by another In this way social survey method is a method considerably free from subjectivity and bias.

(f) It is with the help of social surveys that more and more facts come to light, which were hither to unknown. In every society there are certain hidden problems which do not wish these to come to light or because these are not known to society. Surveys reveal these facts and ones these are focused, new theories are expounded and in this way the whole social science community gains.

To Sum Up:

1. It is one of widely used method and it has universal application.
2. Social surveys are based on actual observations.

3. Surveys have proved their usefulness in leading to the formulation of nypothesis.
4. A survey brings the researcher in a position to come face to face with the realities of life and see things personally.
5. Survey method is very useful in testing the validity of many theories.
6. The survey method avoids the possibility of personal biases.
7. It saves time since data are collected analyzed more quickly.
8. Above all, sampling errors can be calculated.

DISADVANTAGES OF SOCIAL SURVEY METHOD

The social survey method though so useful as seen in the earlier paragraphs, it is not without its share of limitations and problems.

(a) Firstly it is the problem of resources, both human and economic. Heavy amounts are needed for getting every survey conducted. It also involves a lot of manpower in the form of trained investigators, field workers etc. Further, manpower is also needed at the administrative level for co-ordination and technical staff for analysis and so on.

(b) Then another difficulty is lack of uniformity in the collection of data. When so many persons are on the field, obviously each one will give his own interpretation to the terms used in the data collection schedule and when there is no uniformity there is bound to be variance. Thus, there is room for individual bias and eliminating it becomes an difficult task later on.

(c) Survey method of research is time consuming.

(d) In spite of good planning it is a matter of common knowledge that when large scale surveys are taken up many unanticipated difficulties creep in sometimes these problems may be easily solved and sometimes these become really serious and the research work suffers.

(e) Data collected with the help of survey method can become dependable and reliable only when two basic conditions are met. One is that the investigators who are given the responsibility of collecting data should be trained and they should be persons of with integrity, and responsibility. On the other another pre-ponds should be prepared to cooperate and come out with correct information. Both these are really great hurdles. It is difficult to find out trained and willing field investigators because usually the investigators go to the field for the sake of earning bread and not with the sense of involvement. Similarly in large surveys it is not possible to have willing respondents. May be that a substantial percentage of people are forthcoming to cooperate with the researcher, but vast majority is not research conscious and as such not or less a futile exercise and extent of reliability becomes uncertain.

(f) Still another difficulty is that either the results are to be generalized or localized. If survey of a particular local area is conducted then obviously the results obtained will be applicable to that particular area.. On the other hand, when survey is spread to a vast area then the results become too general and not of much use. In this way, in both cases survey has its own limitations.

(g) Finally, it must be noted that large scale surveys cannot be undertaken and a way out, is to pick samples for the study. If a sample survey is not carefully planned and executed, the inferences drawn may be inaccurate and misleading. Its results may be accurate and applicable to the whole universe if the sample taken is a true representative of the universe which is a very difficult task. When sampling method is used then sampling errors are bound to creep in. In all this the defects of sampling method of social research gets introduced in the study.

(h) Under this method bias may vitiate the result. (W.I. King)

(i) The survey method lacks flexibility.

(j) Survey method is only useful for current problems and is not suitable for the problem that requires the study in the historical retrospect.

Steps of a Social Survey

1. Selection of a problem
2. Preliminary study or pilot study
3. General objective of the study
4. Specific objectives
5. Resources and personnels.

CASE STUDY METHOD

The methods of scientific social research may broadly be divided into two parts: the statistical methods and the case study methods. The statistical methods are based on large scale collection of facts, while case study is based on intensive study of comparatively fewer persons. The case study is more intensive in nature. The field of study is comparatively limited but has more of depth in it. It aims at studying everything about something, rather than something about everything as in the case of statistical methods. It is concerned with everything that is significant in the history or development of the case. In one sense, the case study method is a vertical study. It delves into the past, brings the description up to the present and tries to predict the future. In another, it is a horizontal study, seeking to find out and establish the inter-relationship between the reference unit and the rest of the social or economic system. The case study is thus both a longitudinal and latitudinal study. It has a historical approach and its object is to give a picture of the living, throbbing organism that a social unit is. This calls for an inter-disciplinary approach.

Definition

Pauline V. Young: "Case study is a method of exploring and analyzing of life of a social unit be that a personal, a family, institution, cultural group or even entire community." It is "a comprehensive study of a social unit a person, a group, a social institution, a district or a community."

F.L. Whitney: "Case study is a complete analysis and report of the status of an individual subject with respect as a rule to specific phases of his total personality."

Goode and Hatt: "Case study is a way of organizing social data so as to preserve the unitary character of the social object being studied. Expressed somewhat differently it is an approach which views any social unit as a whole."

Yang Hsin Pao: "Case study method may be defined as small inclusive and intensive study of an individual in which investigator brings to bear all his skills and methods or as a systematic gathering of enough information about a person to permit one to understand how he or she functions as unit of society."

H. Odum: "The case study method is a technique by which individual factor whether it be an institution or just an episode in the life of an individual or group is analyzed in its relationship to any other in the group."

Case study method is concerned with everything that is significant in the history or development of the case. The purpose is to understand the life cycle or an important part of the life cycle of an individual unit.

With the above definitions, we can deduce the following characteristics of case study method :

(a) Unit of study may be an individual, a family, an institution a culture group or an entire community. It may also be an abstract thing like a set of relationship or processes, viz,, family crisis, adjustment disease, etc., therefore, it is clear that a wide variety of unit may be selected for the purpose of study and the size of the unit may be fairly large to cover an entire nation or a community. Each unit is taken as a whole.

(b) Case study aims at deep and detailed study of the unit. According to Goode and Hatt, it is an approach which views any social unit as a whole. This is where the case study differs fundamentally from the statistical method. In case of Statistical methods we take a certain aspect of the problem and collect material about it, as if each individual set of behaviour were complete in itself and separate from the life of the person as a whole.

(c) The selected unit is studied intensively.

(d) The approach happens to be qualitative and not quantitative.

(e) It is made to know the mutual inter-relationship of causal factors.

(f) In the case of Case Study, the life of the individual or family is indivisible whole and we cannot arrive at the real truth behind any behaviour unless we have studied the life as a whole in all its aspects. The case method connects the thoughts and attempts to keep together units and their characteristics which are relevant to the scientific problem being investigated. The Unit is taken as representative of a group and only those aspects of his life are studied and that are relevant to the problem under study which are in conformity with his status as a representative unit of society or group.

(g) The characteristics of a good case study include an adequate data which is valid, continuous, carefully synthesized, confidential which should be useful for fellowship. An adequate case history clarifies epistemological relationship, resolves controversial points, uncovers illogical thinking and misinformation and aids in the differentiation between functional and organic complaints.

Distinction Between Case Study Method and Statistical Method

"Statistical technique depends upon the reduction of data to quantitative terms in order to yield totals, averages and correlations; the case study technique seeks data in terms of processes which, for the most part, cannot be stated numerically. The statistician selects certain specific factors involved in social institutions and manipulates them so as to discover the relation between the several variables. The case student examines single situation, persons, groups, institutions as complex wholes in order to identify types and process." (Pauline Young)

History of Case Study Method

Case study had its beginning in the middle of the 19th C, Charles Booth, the author of "Life and Labour of the People of London", adopted the basic methods of case study – participant observation, interview, questionnaire and the use of the secondary data. Fredrick Le Play of France was his French counterpart. They were followed by Rowntree, Dr. Bowley in England, Paul Kellog (Pittsburg Survey) and Jacob Rii (How the Other Half Live, 1890) in the U.S.A. who developed this method. Under-developed countries too resorted to case study method in several spheres of social and economic activities. One of the earlier case studies in India was Gilbert Slater's "Some South Indian Villages". The Research Programme Committee of the Planning Commission sponsored a large number of case studies in the 1950s, e.g., Economic Survey of Chennai City, Beggar Surveys in Hyderabad, Prostitution in Mumbai and Industrial Case Studies in Tamil Nadu State.

Following are the **basic assumptions** underlying Case Study:

(a) **Totality of the being:** The first fundamental assumption of the case study is that of a unit is indivisible whole and cannot be studied piecemeal and in fragments. In order to study the behaviour of an individual at any particular time it is not enough to study his situation at the particular time alone. We must have his whole life history, his background before we can really explain his behaviour at the particular time. It is because of this basic assumptions, that the unit has to be studied in its wholeness.

(b) The unit selected is the representative of the group.

(c) Uniformity in the basic human nature.

(d) **Underlying unity:** In the face of apparent diversity among different units there is an underlying units. A particular unit has its uniqueness but it is not different from other units in all respects. It is also representative of a group and can be studied as a type rather than a pure individual. This underlying unity makes it possible for us to apply the inference drawn from the unit or group of units to the group as a whole. It is because of this assumption that study of a particular unit has any fruitful application in the prediction and control of the social phenomena.

(e) **Complexity of social phenomena:** Social phenomenon is not only a total whole it is very complex also. A greater part of man's life is subjective unknown and incapable of observation. The understanding of human nature and his action requires much deeper probe and a keen insight. A sympathetic study of a human behaviour is possible only through case study.

(f) The assumption of studying the natural history of the unit concerned.

(g) **Influence of time:** Social phenomena are influenced by time also. In order to find out the real motives behind any action, we have to study the problem in its historical perspective. Without the knowledge of past history the study would remain incomplete and would yield results that would be untrue. It is because of this influence of time that under case study we examine the unit over full cycle of time.

Source of Case Data

The sources of case data may be divided into two parts:

(i) Personal Documents

(ii) Life History.

(i) **Personal Documents:** Most of the people keep diaries, write their autobiographies or memories. These personal documents contain the description of the remarkable events of the life of the narrator as well as his reaction towards them. They may also contain the description of even those events in which he has played his part only as a witness of a distant spectator. These documents are self-revealing records which intentionally or unintentionally yield direct information regarding the structure, dynamics and functioning of author's mental life. These personal documents, although sufficiently subjective in nature are nevertheless highly important for social research. Diaries are mostly written for self satisfaction and the writer is not likely to distort facts deliberately. Such document's may be written for general purpose and later on used by the researcher. According to Pauline Young, 'Personal documents represent continuity in experience which helps to illuminate the writer's personality. Social relations and philosophy of life often expressed in objective reality or subjective appreciation'. They are very helpful in studying the personality of the writer and his reactions to different circumstances of life.

(ii) **Life History:** Life History is the study of various events of respondent's life together and it finds their social significance. It is in this way that life history differs from the pure historical narrative of facts. While the pure narrative aims narrating the facts only, life history aims at revealing the meaning and significance of those events in the text of motivating factors of social life. It is the combination of facts and inference. Life History data is generally gathered through prolonged interviews with the respondent's use of any written material available about his life and the analysis of the facts so collected in order to draw a valid generalization from them.

Besides the above two methods, various other methods may also be adopted. According to Pauline Young, the other methods may include from simple verification methods like periodical conferences, dramatic productions, observation and post experimental interviews, to more complicated processes like experimental studies, a wide range of test including hypnotic tests, test of ability, test of aesthetic appreciation, emotional conditioning, social reaction to frustration, imagination, productivity, psychological insight etc.

Steps Involved in Case Study

(i) Selection of cases and identification of situations.

(ii) Collection and recording of data.

(iii) Interpretation of data.

(iv) Report writing.

Importance of Case Study

(i) Case Study helps in formulating valid hypothesis. When various cases are thoroughly studied and carefully analyzed, the researcher can arrive at various generalizations, which may be developed into useful hypothesis.

(ii) Case Study is useful in framing questionnaire, schedule or other forms. If a questionnaire is drafted after case study, we can know the peculiarities of the group as well as individual units, the type of response likely to be available.

(iii) Case Study is helpful in stratification of the sample. By studying the individual units thoroughly we can put them in definite classes or types.

(iv) Through Case Study it is possible to locate cases. Deviant cases are those units that behave against the proposed hypothesis. A general tendency is to ignore them, but for scientific analysis they are very important.

(v) The Case Study enlarges the range of personal experience of the researcher. In Statistical methods, generally a narrow range of topic is selected and the researcher's knowledge is limited to the particular aspect only. In case study, the whole range of subject's life is studied and the range of knowledge is naturally enlarged. The researcher gets an intimate knowledge of many other aspects.

(vi) The Case Study helps to find the significance of the recorded data within the individual and later on within the life of the classes of individuals. The researcher comes into contact with different classes of people. He watches their life and hears their experiences.

(vii) It produces new ideas and fresh suggestions

(viii) It helps in formulating a sound hypothesis

(ix) It may also help in exploring new areas of research.

Limitation of Case Study Method

Case study method has also subject to certain criticisms:

(i) **Overconfidence of the researcher:** In the case of Statistical studies, the researcher knows his limitations. He knows fully well that he has studied only one aspect of the problem and while proceeding his research, he would be very cautious, In the case of Case study, the researcher studies each unit in its complete dimensions. The researcher begins to feel as if he knows everything about the unit and needs no further enlightenment about it. Practically it is not so.

(ii) **Unsystematic:** The Case method is Unsystematic. No controls are exercised upon the informant or the researcher. The data collected in this way is generally incapable of verification and the generalization drawn from it are also not very accurate.

(iii) **This method is generalized:** Generalizations are drawn from few cases. What the researcher thinks to be the common trait of human nature may be personal peculiarity of the subject and, therefore, applicable to particular person only.

(iv) **Error may creep in due to inaccurate observation:** Due to inaccurate observation, there is scope for errors. There may be errors in reporting, failure of the memory, it describes what is more imaginary than real.

(v) **Too costly affair:** For the Case study too much of time and money should be spent.

(vi) **Not scientific:** The researcher instead of finding some scientific explanation for a particular phenomena, he tries to find some common sense explanation which is purely based on intuition. Such things could not be relied upon.

(vii) Case study does not provide universal, impersonal and common aspects of a phenomenon.

(viii) The case study method is not in itself a scientific method at all, but merely a first step in scientific procedure because it is qualitative in character and is not very useful for quantitative studies.

EXPERIMENTAL METHOD

Experimental research examines what will happen when certain variables are carefully controlled or manipulated. It examines cause and effect relationship, e.g., comparison of output between the uses of traditional and HYV seeds of paddy; behaviour of radio listeners and others regarding family planning practices. Experiment has been regarded as the sole basis of scientific method for fairly long time and it was on this basis that social sciences were denied the place of science. The use of this method has primarily been made in the physical sciences where the subject matter can be given the laboratory treatment under controlled conditions.

Experimental method which for a fairly long time remained the exclusive domain of the physical scientists, is gradually finding favour with social sciences as well. This has been made possible by the scientific equipment that has been made available to the social scientists, and also refinements in the tools of analysis through researches in the methodology.

Definitions

V.H. Bedkar: "Experimental method implies a controlled observation of a succession of events. The aim is to search for causal connection."

Jahoda and Others: "Social experiment is a method of testing hypothesis."

E. Greenwood: "An experiment is the proof of a hypothesis which seeks to hook up two factors into a casual relationship through the study of contrasting situations which have been controlled on all factor except the one of interest, the latter being either the hypothetical case or the hypothetical effect."

Festinger: "The essence of an experiment may be described as observing the effect on a department variable of the manipulation or an independent variable."

"The basic factor in case of experimental method is the control over the subject of study and manipulation of the independent variable to study its effect upon the dependent variables."

"In the narrowest sense only pure laboratory experiments are to be included in the category of experiments, as the experimenter exercises absolute control over the subject and is in a position to introduce stimulus in the varying degree while keeping other variable stable."

The process of examining the truth of a statistical hypothesis, relating to some research problem is known as an experiment. For example, the researcher can conduct an experiment to examine the usefulness of a certain newly developed drug. There are two types of experiments namely absolute experiment and comparative experiment. If the researcher wants to determine the impact of the fertilizer on the yield of a crop, it is a case of absolute experiment. But if the researcher wants to determine the impact of one fertilizer as compared to the impact of some other fertilizer, then the experiment is termed as comparative experiment. A research in which the independent variable is manipulated is termed "experimental hypothesis-testing research."

Types of Experiments

Social experiments may be divided into various classes according to the type of setting nature and extent of control and the technique adopted for manipulating the variable.

Five types of Experiments have been suggested by Greenwood:

(i) **Trial and error experiment:** Under this method the researcher does not prepare a structured plan of study. He prepare a hypothesis and tries to test it on actual social conditions wherever they may be found. As the study is not rigidly planned his technique will undergo a constant modifications in the light of experience. For example he may start his studies on a small group; but later on finding that it was unsuitable may enlarge it or change it altogether. This type of experiment may not be called scientific and it is a waste of time.

(ii) **Controlled observational study:** This includes observation of the phenomena under controlled conditions and it is almost like laboratory type experiment. Under this method a stimulus is provided to the subject and changes are observed to find out the casual effect of the stimulus.

(iii) **Natural experiment:** This is also called as Field Experiment. The Experiment is conducted in the natural setting, but it is different from the field of study or field observation. In the case of field experiment, we try to manipulate the independent variable while in the case of field study. We simply observe the phenomena taking place without any kind of manipulation.

Abraham Kaplan narrates the following types of experiments:

(a) Methodological,

(b) Pilot study,

(c) Heuristic,

(d) Fact finding,

(e) Boundary (designed to fix the range of application of laws),

(f) Simulation (experiments on model),

(g) Nomological (aimed at establishing a law, proving or disproving some hypotheses),

(h) Theoretical, and

(i) Illustrative.

(iv) **Ex-ante and Ex-post-facto technique (Before and after approach)/ Evaluation study:** This is a method that helps to carry the ceteris paribus assumption of the abstract science to the field investigation in applied economics. For instance, in the Benefit-Cost Evaluation of the Cauvery Mettur Project, the object was to estimate the benefit accruing from irrigation. There are two ways of doing it.

Before and after approach is possible if there is a bench-mark study of the command area before waters were released. If so, a current survey conducted in the area after a period of years will furnish data for comparison. The difference between the agricultural inputs and output, and other incomes at both the points of time will give an estimate of the benefits, with due adjustment to changes in prices. This is also called ex-ante and ex-post approach. This is not quite a satisfactory techniques since in the intervening period, various forces could have come into operation and other things would not have remained equal. It is not possible to calculate the impact of these extraneous forces. The technique is used to study the varying influence of two identical factors. Suppose it is proposed to study the influence of Tamil and English education upon future adjustable in life, we shall take an equal number of students in each group keeping in mind that other variables like age, status, intelligence etc., should be matched in both cases. After about 15 years, we shall try to locate those persons and see how they are placed in life. The difference between the two may be attributed to the nature of education received.

(v) **Laboratory experiment:** Festinger defines: Laboratory experiment 'as one in which the investigator creates a situation with the exact conditions he wants to have and in which he controls some manipulated variables.' Laboratory research is meant for small group study of random behaviour which makes use of audio-visual recording devices, use of observation, etc.

The major difference between field experiment and laboratory experiment is that of the nature of setting and degree of control. A field experiment is studied in the natural setting with control over independent variables, for a laboratory experiment the setting is artificially created. For, example, if we make an experiment with the college students in the college itself it would be field experiment, but if we create a small class room and experiment upon it, it will be laboratory experiment. In a laboratory experiment, the phenomena is artificially created and is naturally subject to greater control and manipulation.

Difficulties of Social Experiments

Following are the various difficulties that the experimenter has to face in conducting an experiment:

(i) **Difficulties in setting:** The major difficulty in the case of social experiment is in finding out proper setting. In the case of laboratory experiment, the setting has to be created and it is not always possible. There are many social phenomena which cannot be enacted in the laboratory under created conditions. Even where the experiment has to be conducted in the natural setting there is the problem of finding out the place where the phenomena is found insufficiently pure form to follow observation.

(ii) **Difficulties of co-operation:** Human beings who form the subject matter of social experiment are not so easy to be manipulated. They work according to their free will and their willing co-operation with the experiment is necessary. There is a condition which is not always present and lack of interest makes active co-operation difficult. At times even when co-operation is forthcoming from one group, it may not be available from the other group, particularly when two groups are opposed to each other. Even when the co-operation is available it may not be unqualified.

(iii) **Difficult of control:** For successful experiment it is necessary that all other causative factors except the one under study must be strictly unchanged and the particular variable may be vibrated gradually. This is very difficult. The difficulty is mainly created by complexity of social phenomena, its dynamic nature and independence of human behvaiour.

The social phenomenon has a tendency to move secularly. It is not static and therefore, very difficult to control. It is also affected by a number of outside conditions and it is not possible either to control them or to insulate the experimental group entirely from the outside influence. For example, production in the factory may be affected not only by the conditions prevailing inside the factory but also general economic and political conditions in the country, which are impossible to control especially when the experiment has to be conducted for a long time. Independence of human action is another difficulty of control. The very knowledge of the fact that a person is being watched sometimes leads him to behave abnormally.

Validity of Results

Now the question before us is whether the results obtained are practical or whether they are purely hypothetical. The main argument against experimental method in this regard is that chances of its application are rather very dim. The degree of manipulation of independent variable presupposes that the unit of study must be a small and the experiment must be confined over a short period to avoid the influence of confounding factors. Suppose an experiment is conducted upon a small group of labour and it is known that the greater the degree of freedom of work the better is their output. This result is true of the particular group and unless the group itself is representative, the formula cannot be applied with certainty everywhere.

Human behaviour is not governed by particular cause but by total situation as a whole. Therefore, we cannot predict with certainty that freedom of work will increase output in a given quantity. The uncertainty of practical application at times leads to grave doubts about the validity of experimental method. Once we have known with certainty the effect of different causative factors separately and conjunction with other factors, we shall be in a position to predict the results fairly and accurately.

Advantages of Experimental Method

(i) **It determines cause and effect relationship:** The Experimental Method permits the determination of cause and effect relationship more clearly than any other methods. For example, we can say that higher wages and higher output go together, but we cannot say whether higher wages have caused higher output or vice versa: Unless the causes and effect are clearly located, it is not possible to control the phenomena which is the primary practical objective of any research.

(ii) **It is more precise and accurate:** Compared to any other method, the Experimental method is precise and accurate. Since the variable under study is manipulated leaving others unchanged we can locate with, precision the effect of varying degree of stimulus. For example, we can find out precisely the effect of varying degree of freedom of work upon output. A complete freedom of work may result in the fall in production rather than a rise in it. By knowing the effect of varying degree of freedom we can fix up norms of the degree of freedom when the production is highest.

(iii) **Experimental method is the best for testing hypothesis:** Casual observation may help in the formulation of a hypothesis but it is only through experimental method that it can be tested and verified. Testing of hypothesis requires a study of relationship under varied conditions which is possible only under experimental method.

(iv) **Universally acclaimed as scientific method:** Its use in social setup has been limited only because of the difficulties presented by social phenomena and out of lack of knowledge of it rather than due to any defect in the system itself. As our knowledge of the social phenomena increases, we shall be in a position to make increasing use of experimental method.

INFORMATION SYSTEM RESEARCH (ISR)

Europe and America have played a major role in starting the Information System and Research. In Europe and the U.K. in particular, we an point to the mid-1980s, when academicians like David Avison and Guy Fitzgerald from the department of computer science and management, respectively, pondered over the nature of information system, which at the time was in essence applied computing or data processing. By the mid-1960s, the scope of applied computing in organizations was expanded to management levels, and this introduced the concept of MIS (Davis, 1999). The IS Journal within the decade ending 2001 has started accepting papers based on case studies, action research, hermeneutics, critical thinking, agency theory, speech – act – theory, postmodernist theory, grounded theory, feminist theory, personal construct theory and phenomenological research (Avision et al. 2001, p. 14).

ACTION RESEARCH

This is a recent classification. This type of research is conducted through direct action. The actual study may consist of a number of phases – base-line survey, systematic action, periodical assessment, etc. A good example of action research is a study of test marketing. Even in the case of industrial products, machinery and consumer durables, the action research method is used, when, instead of distributing the product, demonstration is made as a part of action research. It is research through launching of a direct action with the objective of obtaining workable solutions to the given problems. Prediction form of hypothesis is more useful in action research studies.

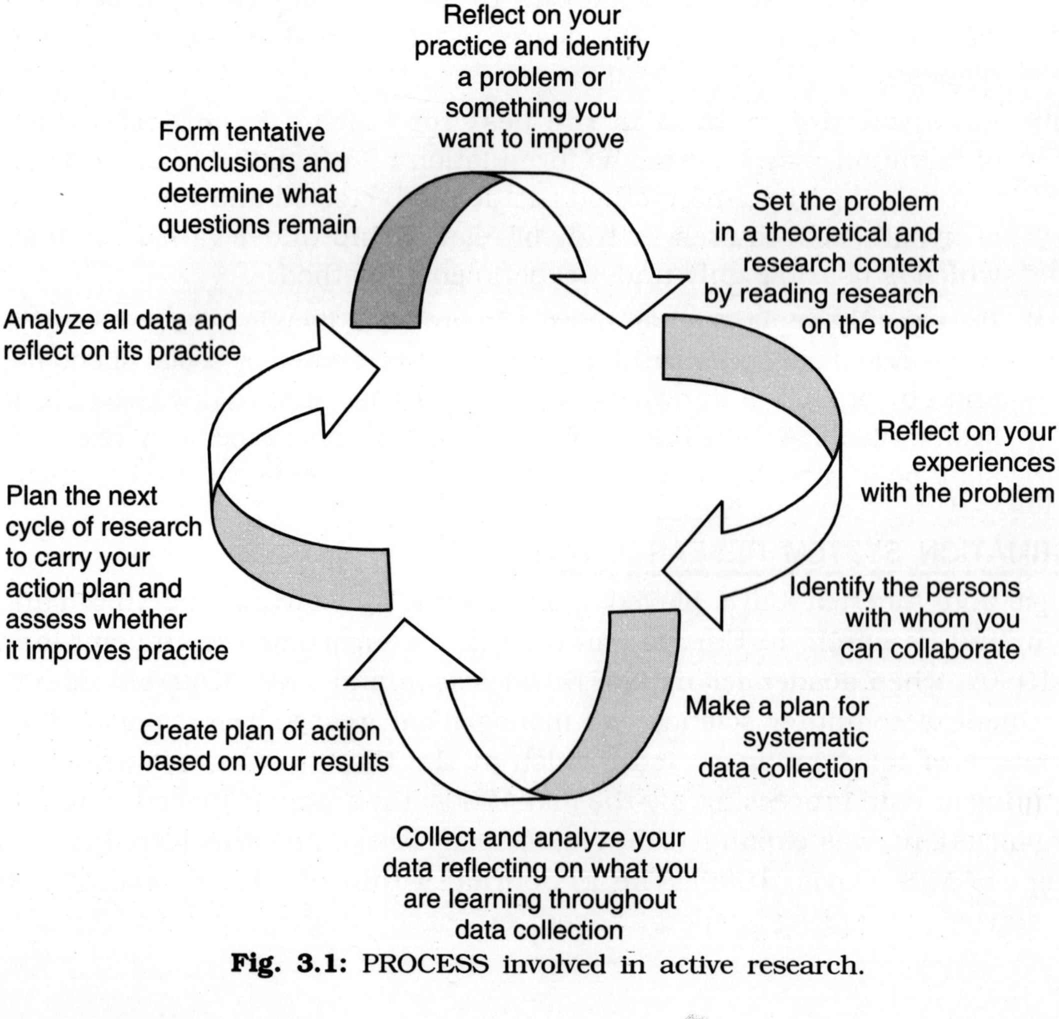

Fig. 3.1: PROCESS involved in active research.

BUSINESS GAME

It is a more improved version of the role played. A game is played in different situations, each situation covering a particular operating and a strategic decision. For example, the participants are divided into groups, each group representing an independent firm in the same industry. The participants are exposed to a number of strategic and operational decisions, covering all the functional areas. At the end of all the situations, the group that shows the best performance is adjudged the best decision-maker.

EVALUATION RESEARCH

Evaluation aims at determining the effects of the operation of a specified variable in quantitative terms. It is a product of developmental programming which has been adopted on a very large scale in the recent years. It is primarily directed to evaluate the performance of the developmental projects and other economic programmes that have already been implemented. Evaluation is held to mean comprehensive concept of measurement and it is because of this definition of evaluation that project evaluation has become frequent in the recent years. The cost-benefit analysis and the evaluation of the various planning and development projects belong to this category. While carrying out the evaluation research a researcher can scientifically look into the performance of the project in relation to the objective that has been laid out and in line with the processes that had been recommended for its implementation.

Types of Evaluation Research:

(i) Concurrent Evaluation

(ii) Periodic or Phasic Evaluation

(iii) Terminal Evaluation

(iv) Field Evaluation.

(i) **Concurrent Evaluation:** It is a continuing process of an inspection of the project that has been launched. Evaluation goes on side by side with the implementation of a project. This type of research not only evaluates the performance but also stimulates it and gives direction and control as and when possible.

(ii) **Periodic/Phasic Evaluation:** It takes place at different stages (phases) of performance of the project. If, for example, a project has been launched in three different stages, in building up an institutional complex, evaluation is conducted at the completion of each stipulated stage of the project. It enables us to evaluate the performance of the completed stage and make adjustments in the subsequent stages after keeping in view the failures and success of the previous stage.

(iii) **Terminal Evaluation:** It is the evaluation of the final stage of the project. Here, an overall assessment is made to see how best a project has served the objectives for which it was launched.

(iv) **Field Evaluation:** The following are the types of Field Evaluation Research.

- Case study and life history
- Mass Observation/Participant observation/Non-participant observation
- Personal Interview
- Group Interview
- Questionnaire etc.

In this type of evaluation, tape recorders, photographic techniques, attitude scales, sociometric scales, etc., are used.

CANONICAL CORRELATION (A CHARACTERISTIC ROOT)

A canonical correlation is a form of correlation relating two set of variables. It is the correlation of two canonical (latent) variables, one represents a set of independent variables, the other a set of dependent variables. Each set may be considered a latent variable based on measured indicator variables in its set. The maximum number of canonical correlation between two sets of variables is the number of variables in the smaller set. The canonical correlation is optimized such that the linear correlation between the two latent variables is maximized. Multiple regression is used for many-to-one relationships, canonical correlation is used for many-to-many relationships. Analogous with ordinary correlation, canonical correlation squared is the percent of variance in the dependent set explained by the independent set of variables along a given dimension (there may be more than one). The purpose of canonical correlation is to explain the relation of the two sets of variables, not to model the individual variables. For each canonical variate we can also assess how strongly it is related to measured variables in its own set, or the set for the other canonical variate. Wilks's lambda is commonly used to test the significance of canonical correlation. Canonical correlation finds the linear combination of variables that produces the largest correlation with the second set of variables. This linear combination, or 'root', is extracted and the process is repeated for the residual data, with the constraint that the second linear combination of variables must not correlate with the first one. The process is repeated until a successive linear combination is no longer significant.

Canonical correlation is a member of the multiple general linear hypothesis family and shares many of the assumptions of multiple regression such as linearity of relationships, homoscedasticity (same level of relationship for the full range of the data), interval or near-interval data untruncated variables, proper specification of the model, lack of high multicollinearity, and multivariate normality for purposes of hypothesis testing. It also shares with factor analysis the need to impute label; for the canonical variables based on structure correlations, which function as a form of canonical factor loading; researchers may well impute different labels based on the sanme data.

CONCEPTS OF CANONICAL CORRELATION

(i) **Eigen values:** The eigenvalues as computed by SPSS are approximately equal to the canonical correlation squared. They reflect the proportion of variance explained by each canonical correlation relating two sets of variables, when there is more than one extracted canonical correlation. There is one eigenvalue for each canonical correlation. There will be as many eigen values as there are canonical correlations (roots), and each successive eigen value will be smaller than the last since each successive root will explain less and less of the data.

(ii) **Canonical variable or variate:** It is a linear combination of a set of original variables in which the within-set correlation has been controlled

(iii) **Canonical coefficient (canonical function coefficient or canonical weight):** It is the standardized weights in the linear equation of variables which creates the canonical variables. It is used to assess the relative importance of individual variables' contributions to a given canonical correlation. There will be one canonical coefficient for each original variable in each of the two sets of variables, for each canonical correlation. Thus for the dependent set, if there are five variables and there are three canonical correlations (functions), there will be 15 canonical coefficients in three sets of five coefficients.

(iv) **Canonical factor loadings (structure correlation coefficients):** A structure correlation is the correlation of a canonical variable with an original variable in its set. It is the correlation of canonical variable scores for a given canonical variable with the standardized scores of an original input variable.

MODELLING RESEARCH

A model is an abstraction of reality. Many of the real-life problems of business situations can be formulated as models.

TYPES OF MODELLING RESEARCH

(i) **Symbolic Model:** It is a representation cf the performance measure of the system of interest in terms of its variables. This means that the attributes of a system are related by an equation. Regression equation is an example of symbolic model.

(ii) **Mathemetical Model:** It is mainly operations research model which is aimed to solve complex real-life problems arising in the direction and management of large systems of men, materials, money, and machines in business, industry. And government. Some examples of this model are transportation model, assignment model, linear programming model, separable programming model, inventory model, chance constrained programming model, replacement model, parametric programming model, quadratic programming model, goal programming model, etc. In this mathematical model, one can do any one of the following types of research:

(a) Use of any one or a combination of existing mathematical models to obtain the results of a complex problem.

(b) Development of improved method for each of the mathematical modeling techniques.

Conclusive Research: It tests the hypothesis of a research problem formulated by exploratory research and draws definite conclusion for implementation. It is classified into descriptive research and experimental research.

BRANCH AND BOUND METHOD OF ENUMERATION

It is a curtailed enumeration method. In this method, the creation of certain sub-problems will be curtailed by the usage of a strong lower bound in the case of minimization problem or a strong upper bund in the case of maximization problem.

The branch and bound method employs any one of the following approaches for branching to create sub-problems: (i) Depth first search method and (ii) Breath first search method.

The first method stated above requires less memory space to store the sub-problems. In the second method, one can find the solution quickly in comparison with the first method but it requires lot of memory space to store the sub-problems.

The branching procedure removes the original problem with a set of new sub-problems that are: (i) smaller problems than the original problem, (ii) partially solved version of the original problem, and (iii) Mutually exclusive and collectively exhaustive sub-problems of the original problem.

The branch and bound method should be applied to only small size or moderate size problems. The usage of more and more stronger bound can enhance the size of the problem that can be solved using the branch and bound method.

HEURISTICS

Any method which is used to solve a combinatorial problem near-optimally in finite time is called heuristic. A heuristic can also give the optimal solution on some trials. In general, a method is called heuristic until there is a proof that it will give an optimal solution for all the problems and for all trials on each problem. When the number of sub-problems of a given combinatorial problem grows exponentially with respect to its problem size, it will be difficult to solve any combinatorial problem optimally using exact algorithms, like, census enumeration method, branch and bound method etc., If one can solve a combinatorial problem optimally in finite time using some method, then similar method can be extended to solve all other combinatorial problems in literature. However, it is impossible to solve all the combinatorial problems in literature optimally in finite time. But the practitioners need to solve such problems in finite time to carry out their businesses. Hence, they prefer to solve the combinatorial problems near-optimally in finite time using some suitable method.

SIMULATION

Simulation is an experiment conducted on a model of some system of interest. Consider an example of the queueing system, namely the reservation system of a transport corporation. The elements of the system are booking counters (servers) and waiting customers (queues). Generally, the arrival rate of the customers follows Poisson distribution and the services time follows exponential distribution. If the reservation system has the above combination of distribution, then the queueing model can be used to find the standard results.

Types of simulation: (i) Identity simulation (observing the behaviour of the real world under as many operational configurations as possible to get an insight into system behaviour), (ii) Quasi-identity simulation (aspecs of the real-world system are preserved while some elements whose presence would make the identity simulation impossible are excluded, e.g., simulation of an air attack over a country by its enemy aircraft), (iii) Laboratory simulation (transactions will be carried out over a specified period and then the operating performance of the business will be reviewed), and (iv) Computer simulation (we remove people from the laboratory simulation with a well-designed computer logic and retain other aspects).

Some of the systems on which the simulation experiment can be carried out are:

- Simulation of portfolio mix
- Simulation of labour turnover
- Simulation of labour absenteeism
- Simulation of customers' waiting at bank counters etc.

CHAPTER 4 Research Design

MEANING OF RESEARCH DESIGN

A plan of action prepared by a research scholar for his study is known as research design. Research design is the conceptual structure within which research is conducted; it constitutes the blue print for the collection, measurement and analysis of data. It is the plan, structure and strategy of investigation conceived so as to obtain answers to research questions and control variance. "Research design is a catalogue of the various phases and facts relating to the formulation of a research effort. It is an arrangement of the essential conditions for collection and analysis of data in a manner that aims to combine relevance to the research purpose with economy in procedure (Claire Selltiz). Decision regarding when, where, how much, by what means, concerning an inquiry or a research study constitute a research design. It is a research strategy, An arrangement of conditions for collection and analysis of data in a manner that aims to combine relevance to the research papers with economy in procedure. It constitutes the blue print for the collection and analysis of data in a manner that aims to combine relevance to the research papers with economy in procedure. It constitutes the blue print for the collection, measurement and analysis of data. It is a tentative plan which undergoes many changes as the study progresses. It guides the researcher to progress in the right direction. It gives an outline of the structure and process of the research work. According to Bernard S. Phillips, research design constitutes the blueprint for the collection, measurement and analysis of data.

The research design includes various steps like selection of a research problem, background to the problem, formulation of objective and hypothesis, conceptual clarity, methodology, survey of literature, documentation, data collection, bibliography, testing of the hypothesis, interpretation, presentation and report writing.

In short, research design should have (a) a clear statement of the problem, (b) procedure and techniques to be used for collecting information, (c) the population to be studied, and (d) methods to be adopted in the processing and analysis of data.

CHARACTERISTICS OF A GOOD RESEARCH DESIGN

A good research design must not only be appropriate but must yield results from the research that can be interpret with confidence. Four characteristics of a good research design are identified. However they cannot be considered naturally independent of each other. They are free from bias, free from confounding control of extraneous variables and statistical precision for testing hypothesis.

Free from bias: This means that the data and the statistics computed from them do not vary in any systematic except as expected on the basis of random fluctuations. The differences that appear can be attributed to the independent variable under the study. Bias can enter into the data in a number of ways, including biased assignment of the individuals to the experimental method.

Freedom from confounding: A good research design should eliminate confounding of variables or keeps it to a minimum so that we can separate effects and we can interpret results without confusion. Two or more variables are confounded if their effects cannot be separated. In physics, for example, if there are trainers instead of one trainer and if the students trained in one type of motivation score higher than those of the other two types we will not know whether the higher performance is due to one type or to the trainer. The effects of trainer and type of motivation cannot be separated because each trainer uses only a single type.

Control of extraneous variables: The control of extraneous variables means that the influence of independent variables outside to the purposes of the study are minimized, nullified or isolated. In other-words the variance of such variables is in effect reduced to zero or near zero. There are three ways to control extraneous variables. First, if possible eliminate variable as a variable. For example, if we select only one sex for an experiment then we can be sure that sex cannot be a contributing independent variable. Here, we lose the power of generalization. For instance, if we use only boys in the experiment, we cannot say anything about the relation understudy with girls.

The second method to control extraneous variance is through randomization. Theoretically randomization is the only method of controlling all possible extraneous variables. This does not mean that the groups should be equal in all possible variables. By chance, the groups can be unequal but the probability of their being equal is greater.

The third means of controlling extraneous variables are to build it into the design as an independent variable. For example, if sex is to be controlled, then it can be added as another independent variable.

The fourth way to control extraneous variance is to match subjects. The basic principle is to split a variable into two or more parts, (example high and low intelligence) and then randomize within each level but care should be taken on the subjects which are matched. They should be related to the dependent variable.

Statistical precision for testing hypothesis: Another characteristic of a good a research is that it will provide appropriate data with enough precision to test those hypotheses that required statistical tests. In statistical sense, precision is increased as random (or error) variance is decreased.

The preparation of the research design depends on the following:

- Time available for research.
- Finance available for the purpose.
- Means of obtaining the information.
- Availability and skills of the researcher and his staff.
- Explanation of the way in which selected means of obtaining information will be organized along with the reasoning leading to the selection.

Important Aspects of Research Design

(i) Clear statement of the research problem.

(ii) Procedures and techniques to be used for gathering information.

(iii) The Population to be studied.

(iv) Methods to be used in processing and analyzing data.

The selection of a method and planning of the design in time is the first step in research design. It is a blue-print. It is only tentative. However, it is useful to the extent of laying down a series of guide to keep one headed in the right direction. A good research design should satisfy the following four conditions: objectivity, reliability, validity and generalizability of the findings.

NEED FOR RESEARCH DESIGN

Research design is needed because it facilitates the smooth sailing of the various research operation, thereby making research as efficient as possible, yielding maximal information with minimal expenditure of effort, time and money. Research design stands for advance planning of the methods to be adopted for collecting the relevant data and the techniques to be used in their analysis, keeping in view the objective of the research and the availability of the staff and money. Research design, in fact, has a great bearing on the reliability of the results arrived at and as such constitutes the firm foundation of the entire edifice of the research work. A research design helps the researcher to organize his ideas in a form whereby it will be possible for him to look for flaws and inadequacies In the absence of such a course of action, it will be difficult for critic to provide a comprehensive review of the proposed study.

A good design is often characterized by adjectives like flexible, appropriate, efficient, economical and so on. Generally the design which minimizes bias and maximizes the reliability of the data collected and analyzed is considered a good design. The design which gives the smallest experimental error is supposed to be design. Similarly, a design which yields maximal information and gives an opportunity for considering different aspects of a problem is considered most appropriate and efficient design.

Research design pertains to the following decisions:

(i) What is the study about?

(ii) Where is the study being made?

(iii) What is the type of data required?

(iv) Where can the data be found?

(v) When will the study be carried out?

(vi) What is the period of study?

(vii) What is the sample design?

(viii) What are the techniques of data collection?

(ix) How much material or how many cases will be needed?

(x) How will the data be analyzed?

(xi) In what style will the report be prepared?

Relation Between Problem Formulation and Research Design

The research problem or study may be formulated in different forms. It may be formulated with different purposes. The nature of the research design depends on the way in which the problem is formulated. It may be an explanatory one or descriptive or an historical analysis or hypothesis-testing and accordingly the choice of a research design may be made in case of a particular study.

IMPORTANT CONCEPTS/COMPONENTS RELATING TO RESEARCH DESIGN

Before describing the different research designs, it will be appropriate to explain the various concepts relating to designs so that these may be better and easily understood.

1. **Dependent and independent variables:** A concept which can take on different quantitative values is called a variable. As such the concepts like weight, height, income are all examples of variables. Quantitative phenomena (or the attributes) are also qualified on the basis of the presence or absence of the concerning attribute(s). If one variable depends upon or is a consequence of the other variable, it is termed as dependent variable, and the variable that is antecedent to the dependent variable is termed as an independent variable. For instance, if our heights depend upon age, then height is a dependent variable and age is an independent variable.
2. **Extraneous variable:** Independent variable that are not related to the purpose of the study but may affect the dependent variable are termed as extraneous variables. A study must always be so designed that the effect upon the dependent variable is attributed entirely to the independent variable(s) and not to some extraneous variable or variables.
3. **Control:** The technical term 'Control' is used when we design the study minimizing the effects of extraneous independent variables. In experimental researches the term 'control' is used to refer to restrain experimental conditions.
4. **Confound relationship:** When the dependent variable is not free from the influence of extraneous variable(s) the relationship between the dependent and independent variable is said to be confounded by an extraneous variable(s).
5. **Research hypothesis:** When a prediction or a hypothesized relationship is to be tested by scientific methods, it is termed as research hypothesis. The research hypothesis is a predictive statement that relates an independent variable to a dependent variable. Usually, a research hypothesis must con-

tain, at least one independent and one dependent variable. Predictive statements, which are not to be objectively verified or the relationship that are assumed but not to be tested are not termed research hypothesis.

6. **Experimental and non-experimental, hypothesis – testing research:** When the purpose of research is to test a research hypothesis, it is termed as hypothesis-testing research. it can be of the experimental design or of the non-experimental design. Research in which the independent variable is manipulated is termed 'experimental hypothesis-testing research' and a research in which an independent variable is not manipulated is called 'non-experimental hypothesis-testing research.
7. **Experimental and control groups:** In an experimental hypothesis testing research when a group is exposed to usual conditions, it is termed a 'Control' group but when the group is exposed to some novel or special condition, it is termed an experimental group.

   It is possible to design studies which include only experimental groups or studies which include both experimental and control groups.
8. **Treatments:** The different conditions under which experimental and control groups are put are usually referred to as treatments. If we want to determine through an experiment the comparative impact of three varieties of fertilizers on the yield of wheel, in that case the three varieties of fertilizers will be treated as three treatments.
9. **Experiment:** The process of examining the truth of a statistical hypothesis, relating to some research problem, is known as an experiment. For example, we can conduct an experiment to examine the usefulness of a certain newly developed drug. Experiments can be two types viz. absolute experiment and comparative experiment. If we want to determine the impact of a fertilizer on the yield of a crop, it is a case of absolute experiment but if we want to determine the impact of one fertilizer as compared to the impact of some other fertilizer, our experiment will then be termed as comparative experiment. Often, we undertake comparative experiments when we talk of designs of experiments.
10. **Experimental unit(s):** The pre-determined plots or the blocks, where different treatments are used, are known as experimental units. Such experimental units must be selected (defined) very carefully.

DIFFERENT RESEARCH DESIGNS

Different research designs can be conveniently described if we categorize them as:

1. Research design in case of exploratory research studies.

2. Research design in case of Descriptive research studies.
3. Research design in case of Hypothesis testing research studies.
4. Diagnostic type research design.
5. Experimental type research design.

DESIGN OF EXPLORATORY OR FORMULATIVE STUDIES

The purpose of exploratory studies is to achieve new insights into a phenomenon. The reason for aiming at new insights or ideas is to formulate a more precise problem or to develop hypothesis for further definite research. As such the research design appropriate for such studies must be flexible enough to provide an opportunity for considering different aspects of a problem under study.

(a) **Survey of literature:** It means a review of literature in the pertinent field and in the fields or related social sciences. Hypothesis stated by earlier workers may be reviewed and their usefulness may be evaluated as a bias for further research. It may also be considered whether the already stated hypothesis suggest new hypothesis. In this way the researcher should review and build upon the work already done by others.

(b) **Experience survey:** This is a survey to the people who have had practical experience in the fields of relative social sciences. The object of such survey is to obtain insight into the relationship between variables and new ideas relating to the research problem. The researcher must prepare an interview schedule for the systematic questioning of informants.

(c) **Analysis of "insight stimulating" cases:** It is a fruitful method for suggesting hypothesis for research. It is particularly suitable in areas where there is little experience to serve as a guide. This method consists of an intensive study in the selected instances of the phenomenon in which one is interested.

RESEARCH DESIGN IN CASE OF HYPOTHESIS – TESTING RESEARCH STUDIES

Hypothesis-testing research studies (Generally known as experimental studies) are those where the researcher tests the hypothesis of casual relationships between variables. Such studies require procedures that will not only reduce bias and increase reliability, but will permit drawing inferences about casualty. Usually experiments meet this requirement. The study of experimental deigns has its origin in agricultural research. To day, the experimental designs are used in resources relating to phenomena of several disciplines.

Professor Fisher has enumerated three principles of experimental designs:

(1) The Principle of Replication

(2) The Principle of Randomization

(3) The Principle of Local Control.

According to the Principle of Replication, the experiment should be repeated more than once. Thus, each treatment is applied in many experimental units instead of one. By doing so, the statistical accuracy of the experiments is increased, For example, if we are to examine the two varieties of rice, we may divide the paddy field into two parts and grow one variety in one part and other variety in the other part. We can then compare the yield of the two parts and draw conclusion on that basis. But if we were to apply the principle of Replication to this experiment, then we first divide the field into several parts, grow variety in half of these parts and other variety in the remaining parts. We can then collect the data of yield of the two varieties and draw conclusion by comparing the same. The result so obtained will be more reliable in comparison to the conclusions we draw without applying the principle of Replication. The entire experiment can even be repeated several times for better results.

The principle of Randomization provides protection when we conduct an experiment, against the effects of extraneous factors by randomization. In other words, this principle indicates that we should design or plan the experiment in such a way that the variations caused by extraneous factors can all be combined under the general heading of "chance". For instance, if we grow one variety of rice, say in the first of the half of a field and the other variety is grown in the other half, then, it is just possible that the soil fertility may be different in the first half in comparison to the other half. If this is so, our results would not be realistic. In such a situation, we may assign the variety of rice to be grown in different parts of the field on the basis of some random sampling technique, i.e., we may apply randomization principle and protect ourselves against the effects of the extraneous factors (soil fertility differences in the given case). As such, through the application of the principle of randomization, we can have a better estimate of the experimental error.

The principle of Local control is another important principle of experimental design. Under it the extraneous factor, the known source of variability, is made to vary deliberately over as wide a range as necessary and this needs to be done in such a way that the variability it causes can be measured and hence eliminated from the experiment in a manner that we can perform a two-way analysis of variance, in which the total variability of the data is divided into three components attributed to treatments (varieties of rice in our case), the extraneous factors (soil fertility in our case), and experimental error. In other words, according to the principle of local control, we first divide the field into several homogeneous parts, known as blocks. Blocks are the levels at which we hold an extraneous factor fixed, so that we can measure its contribution to the total variability of the data by means of two-way analysis of variance. In brief, through the principle of local control we can eliminate the variability due to extraneous factor(s) from the experimental error.

MAJOR STEPS IN PREPARING A RESEARCH DESIGN

1. **Title of the Problem:** The title of the problem selected by the research scholar should be brief and precise. He should make it clear on what problem he is concentrating.
2. **Review of Earlier Literature:** Review of literature on the area of research is the preliminary step before attempting to plan the study. It is essential to review all the relevant material connected, and with the problem chosen. It is necessary to show that his work differs with the existing literature. After going through the concerned work, one will get an insight into the problem and thus will be able to formulate a correct plan for his future investigation. According to Bedford A. Fabura, any research study should invariably be preceded by survey of literature for the purpose of getting an insight into the works aready conducted.
3. **Sources of Information to be Tapped:** The sources of information to be tapped vary with the interest of the researcher and the type of his study. The sources are divided into documentary and field sources. The latter include living persons who have been in intimate contact with social conditions and changes over a considerable period of time. These persons are regarded as personal sources or direct sources. Documentary sources of information are those which are contained in the published and unpublished documents, reports, statistics, manuscripts, letters, diaries and so on. These sources are either primary or secondary. Primary source of information include data gathered at first hand (i.e., the responsibility for their complication and promulgation remaining under the same authority) and summaries gathered from primary sources.
4. **Development of Bibliography:** As soon as the consultation of available source is begun, the development of bibliography preferably with annotations should be undertaken. Each reference should appear on a separate card or sheet with last name of the author first, his initials or given name following and then the of the reference, publisher's name and the data of publication.
5. **Nature of Study:** The next step in formulating research design is to ascertain the nature of study, whether it is statistical study, case study or a

comparative study or an experimental study or a combination of these and other types, should be decided. Since research study is complex, the specific nature of study should be determined early and precisely.

6. **Objectives of Study:** The objectives of the research study should be complied in clear cut terms. The objectives, of course differ with the nature of studies and goals to be attained. Some times, hypothesis may be formulated and tested. These should be closely and clearly stated and the relationship to previous research made clear.
7. **Scope of the Study:** It is always better to define and delimit the scope of the study. Once the scope of the investigation is fixed, the researcher will have a definite idea of his study.
8. **Conceptualization of Terms Used:** The research student is required to make his mind clear by defining the meaning attached or wanted to attach to the different terms used in the study.
9. **Socio-Cultural Context of Study:** If the problem under investigation relates to human beings, then, it is necessary to ascertain the socio-cultural behaviour pattern of the persons. It is necessary to understand whether the persons adhere, deviate or even withdraw from them completely. Unless this is ascertained, it is not possible to draw useful conclusions.
10. **Geographical Areas to be Covered:** It is essential to determine the geographical area to be covered in connection with research study. Therefore, the physical boundaries of the area are to be specified in the research design.
11. **Periods of Time to be Covered or Time Dimension of the Study:** In the case of historical studies, it is necessary to determine the period to be encompassed so that exploration of the problem will be made easier and clear. This will help the researcher to attribute the conclusion to the particular period in question.
12. **Dimensions of the Study:** It is necessary to make certain assumptions in every study. Wherever these are made they should be stated clearly. Sometimes certain limitations may have to be imposed while making the study. The limits of the proposed investigation should be clearly mentioned in the research design. New concepts should be defined.
13. **The Basis for Selecting the Data:** The factors of time and cost are usually important considerations in social research. It is more economical and efficient to base studies on samples rather than to study the universe. Instead of studying every case which might be included in an investigation logically, only a small portion is selected for analysis. From this analysis, useful conclusions which are equally applicable to the universe can be drawn. Great

care is to be taken in drawing the same from the universe. The sample must also be of adequate size to produce reliable results.

14. **Techniques of Study:** The next stage in the preparation of a research design is the determination of suitable techniques for collection of the necessary data. Here also the techniques that are normally used will differ on the basis of the nature of study. If the study requires close attention of the researcher, observation method will be used. If the subject matter for the study is scattered over a wider area then "questionnaire" may used for collecting such information. If the subject matter to be collected is spread in a limited area, then the 'Schedule and interview' method may be used for collecting the data. Sometimes these techniques may be used collectively in the collection of data relating to the study.

15. **Formulation of Hypothesis:** It is the starting point of research. It is considered as an essential instrument in research. A researcher is supposed to formulate a clear hypothesis to increase the value of the research study. Mr. Guigan suggested the following criteria to frame a good hypothesis:
    (i) It should have logical simplicity.
    (ii) It must be verifiable.
    (iii) It should be expressed in a quantified form.
    (iv) It must be an adequate answer to the specific problem.
    (v) It must be stated in such a way as to allow it to be refuted.

16. **Selection of Sample:** The investigator has to select a sample from the population/universe.

17. **The Control of Error:** The control of error applies principally to experimental studies. The experiment has to consider what variables are operating in a given situation in the laboratory. It is usually possible to control all variables or source of error. For field studies it is usually possible to control key variables and to randomize others. In both cases the variable and other control need to be described.

18. **Establish the Reliability and Validity of Test Instruments:** It is necessary in empirical studies to establish the reliability and validity of instruments. It is of crucial importance in the analytical literacy study too, to evaluate the data collected. Hence, there is the desirability of consulting primary sources rather than secondary sources of information.

19. **Chapter Scheme and Report Writing:** The preparation of a chapter outline is the least step in planning the thesis/dissertation and it is an useful first step in writing the rough drafts. Some of the headings may need to be changed as the investigator progresses. The final form is determined by the nature of the study itself and by conventions. The number of chapters that the study contains and name of each chapter scheme is the objective of the research

problem. The chapter arrangement must include main finding prominently in independent chapters. The first chapter is usually an introductory one and the last chapter is for the findings, conclusions and suggestions. In between is the body of the research report i.e. dissertation/thesis, which vary according to the study.

ADVANTAGES OF RESEARCH DESIGN

There are many advantages which arise an account of the preparation of research design. They are:

(a) Saves a lot of researcher's time.
(b) Directs him to prepare himself for executing various activities systematically.
(c) Enables resource planning procurement in right time.
(d) Better documentation of the activities while the project is in progress.
(e) Ensure project time schedule.
(f) Instils and builds up confidence in the student.
(g) Provides satisfaction and sense of success from the beginning to the completion of every stage of the project.

EXPERIMENTAL DESIGN

SIMPLE POST-TEST DESIGN

In this design two groups and variables are used. One group is known as the experimental group. The other group is control group. The experimental group is exposed to a 'treatment', which is the independent variable. The control group is not exposed to the treatment. The dependent variable is measured for each group.

Suppose we wanted to test the hypothesis that training imparted to administrators during their service increased their efficiency. In the simple post test design we would randomly assign the subjects administrators to a group that will undergo training and to a group that will not. After the training is over we will measure the efficiency of both the groups and if we find any difference between the two groups in efficiency then it is attributed to the effect of training. Here training is independent variable and efficiency it dependent variable.

This experimental design can be diagrammatically shown as following Table 4.1:

Table 4.1.

Random Assignment	Treatment	Post-treatment Measurement of Dependent Variable
Experimental Group	Yes	Yes
Control Group	No	Yes

PRE-TEST AND POST-TEST DESIGN

In this design there is a pre-test of the dependent variable before the experimental treatment is given. This is the major difference between this design and the previous one.

In the example we used simple post-test design. We did not have any pre-test. But here both the groups are subjected to a pre-test before the experimental group is exposed to treatment. That is to say that the efficiency of both the groups is measured before training is given to the experimental group. After the training is over both the groups are post-tested. That is to say that the efficiency of both the groups is once again measured after the training is over. The design can be diagrammatically represented as follows:

Table 4.2: Pre-test and Post-test Design

Random Assignment	Pre-test	Treatment	Post-Test
Experimental Group	Yes	Yes	Yes
Control Group	No	No	Yes

This design has two more advantages than the simple post-test design. Firstly, the effect of extraneous factors can be understood by measuring the change in the control group. Secondly, an analysis of covariance is possible by using the pre-test scores. Analysis of co-variance is more effective than a simple difference between post-test scores.

The Solomon Four-group Design

This design is a combination of the two equivalent group designs previously described (the simple post-test design and the pre-test-post-test design). In this design two experimental groups and two control groups are used. One group is given the pre-test treatment, and a post-test. A second group is given the treatment, and a post-test, but no pre-test. A third group is given a pre-test and post-test. The design can be diagrammatically shown as follows:

Table 4.3: Test Design

Random Assignment	Pre Test	Treatment	Post Test
Experimental group 1	Yes	Yes	Yes
Experimental group 2	No	Yes	Yes
Experimental group 3	Yes	No	Yes
Experimental group 4	No	No	Yes

NON-EXPERIMENTAL DESIGNS

In these designs only a single group is used and the researcher has no control over the application of the test treatment or independent variable. A few important non-experimental designs are described below:

Pre- and Post-test design involves only one group. No control group is used in this design. The one group that is used is given a pre-test, a test treatment, and a post-test. It is assumed that any change in the dependent variable is due to the test treatment. It cannot be ascertained whether the change in the dependent variable was due to the experimental factor. Neither it would be possible to check for pre-test effects.

For example, suppose that we measured the level of political awareness for a group of voters, conducted a orientation course in political matters, re-measured their political awareness level, and then observed that the level of political awareness increased. Are we justified if we concluded that the orientation in political matters was mainly responsible for the increase in political awareness level? We will not be justified because we do not know would have happened if no orientation was given to them. The increase in the level of political awareness could have been result of any number of factors.

Interrupted Time Series Design

Interrupted Time Series Design is an improvement over the pre-test, post-test design. In this design, the researcher establishes trends in the dependent variable by taking measures of the dependent variable before and after the treatment. After establishing trends (either linear or cyclical) the researcher introduces or observes the experimental stimulus. A change in direction of the dependent variable away from the established trend may indicate that the test stimulus has had an effect.

Cross Sectional Design

In this design measurement of the independent variable and the dependent variable are taken at the same point in time. The measurement of the independent variable is used to construct quasi-experimental and quasi-control groups that have naturally occurred and the measurement of the dependent variable are used to assess the differences between the quasi-experimental and quasi-control groups.

For example to test the hypothesis that "those who have high level of political awareness participate more in political activity", we may divide the universe (people) into groups with varying levels of political awareness. We can have one group with no political awareness (quasi-control group) and the others (quasi-experimental group) for observation. The political awareness levels for each of these groups could be measured and contrasted to assess the impact of political awareness on their participation.

Panel Study Design

It is a cross-sectional design that introduces the element. It involves taking measurements of the variables of interest of the researcher on the same units of analysis at several points in time. The measurements of independent and dependent variables are made at the same time. But for this both the panel study and the cross-sectional study are similar. The researcher has no control over which subjects are exposed to the experimental stimulus. In the example we used for explaining the pre test design, we took measurements only after the orientation in political awareness was given. But in the panel study, measurements are taken before and after the orientation are given. Thus in the panel study the researcher waits for the orientation and then create the experimental and control groups. This design helps the researcher reach conclusion with more confidence.

Case Study Design

This involves the observation of one or a few cases of a phenomenon. It is a non experimental design because the researcher has no control over the events under investigation.

CHAPTER 5

Hypothesis

MEANING OF HYPOTHESIS

Hypo means less than and 'thesis' means a generally held view. It is a supposition the validity of which remains to be tested. It is an assumption or proposition whose tenability is to be tested. Ordinarily hypothesis means a mere assumption or some supposition to be proved or disproved. A hypothesis may be formulated in verbal or mathematical form. But for a researcher, hypothesis is a formal question that he intends to resolve. In this sense hypothesis may be defined as a proposition or a test of proposition set forth as an explanation for the observed phenomenon. A hypothesis is a statement temporarily accepted as true in the light of what is, at the time, known about a phenomenon, and it is employed as a basis for action in the search of new truth. A hypothesis is a tentative statement, based on theory or on a cursory examination of a sample or limited amount of data. To make the meaning of hypothesis more clear, let us consider the definitions of experts and the way they have understood the meaning of the term.

A hypothesis is as tentative answer to a question. It should be reasonable, consistent with known facts or theories, stated in such a way that it can be tested and found to be probably true or probably false, stated in the simplest possible terms.

The research hypothesis is a tentative answer to question. It is important that the hypothesis be formulated before data are gathered for an unbiased investigation. Additional hypothesis can be formulated after data are collected provided they are tested on the basis of new data.

George A. Lundberg: A hypothesis is a tentative generalization, the validity of which remains to be tested. In its most elementary stage, the hypothesis may be a mere hunch, guess, imaginative data which becomes the basic for action or investigation.

William C. Emory: When proposition are formulated or empirically tested, they are called hypothesis. Propositions are combined of concepts designated by statements that may be judged true or false, if they refer to observable phenomena.

M.H. Gopal: A tentative solution posed on a cursory observation of known and available data adopted provisionally to explain certain events and to guide in the investigation of others. It is, in fact, a possible solution to the problem.

Fred N. Kerlinger: A conjectural statement of the relation between two or more variables. Hypothesis are always in declarative sentence from and they relate either generally or specially variables to variables.

Goode and Hatt: Define it as a proposition which can be put to test to determine its validity.

Webster's dictionary defines hypothesis as "a proposition condition, or principle which is assumed perhaps without belief in order to draw out its logical consequences and by this method to test its accord with facts which are known or may be determined". George A. Lundberg defines hypothesis as "a tentative generalization, the validity of which remains to be tested". In its most elementary stage the hypothesis may be hunch, the basic for action or investigation. "It is a proposition", say Goods and Hatt, "which can be put to test to determine its validity". These definitions suggest that hypothesis is a conjectural statement of relationship between two or more variables. However, hypothesis is not theory though it is related to it. As W.H. George has put it that theory is an elaborate hypothesis. It is an assumption of proposition whose tenability is to be tested. It is a supposition the validity of which remains to be tested.

A survey of the above viewpoints highlights the fact that hypothesis is a tentative proposition, based on observation of certain occurrences or happenings. It stands to be modified or corrected during the process of investigation demand, if the facts discovered in the course of investigation demand it so.

EXAMPLES OF HYPOTHESIS

To make the student understand better the concept of hypothesis, the following tentatives are given:

(i) A person interested in studying the frequent mishaps in case of newly married women, may formulate his hypothesis like this: the main reason for frequent death in case of newly married women is the non-payment of dowry.

(ii) Similarly, it was reported once in newspaper that about 500 deaths of young women occurred due to accidents. A researcher after going through the relevant information may formulate a tentative hypothesis as the deaths among young women occurred during 1988 in Delhi are not accidents, in fact they are murders committed by husbands and in-laws.

(iii) Leaving side the sociological problems and turning to the propositions in the areas of commerce and management we may formulate as below.

(a) The main reason for sickness among large scale industries is dishonesty and defective financial management by the management.

(b) Traditional investment patterns that are prevailing among the people in the country are responsible for low capital information.

(c) High taxation rates in India are having adverse impact on saving and investment.

(d) Sales growth is directly correlated to the expenditure on advertisement.

(e) Imprudent management of working capital has been the lone cause for poor or inadequate returns in public enterprises.

(f) Unionism prevailing in certain regions is the major cause for non-setting up of industries.

(g) Many factories in India are flouting the provisions of Factories Act, 1948 and thus liable for legal action.

(h) Despite the continued government preaching in curbing concentration of economic power, it has been on the increase, thus, resulting in the failure of legal and non-legal measures.

(i) Government's apathy is the root cause for non-development of small and village industries in India.

(j) Liberal bank credit was strong reason for inventory accumulation in Indian enterprises.

(k) Government's industrial policies have been responsible for structural retrogression in Indian industry since mid-sixties.

REQUIREMENTS OF A SOUND HYPOTHESIS

(i) A hypothesis should clearly specify the dependent and independent variables. For example, income and prices are the independent variables and fertility and area under the crops are the dependant variables.

(ii) The raisondetre for the relationship should be made clear.

(iii) The hypothesis should be capable of being tested by the known techniques of research.

(iv) The hypothesis should be stated briefly and crisply avoiding verbiage.

(v) It must have the simplest of assumptions and smallest number of basic concepts.

FORMULATION OF A WORKING HYPOTHESIS

Going hand in hand with the selection of a research problem is the formulation of a suitable hypothesis. The most difficult exercise which the researcher is required to undergo in the research activity is the formulation of hypothesis. Since the direction of the study is determined by the way the hypothesis are formulated, it assumes further significance. If the researcher is able to formulate a usable hypothesis, much of his problems can be deemed to have been solved, but the problem lies in the fact that what is to be accepted, what is not to be accepted, what facts to be considered, all become a problem to the researcher. It is obvious that hypotheses may have been developed on the basis of pure assumption, observation, shrewd guess or profound hunch. When such is the basis for hypothesis formulation, the formulation of testable hypothesis proves to be really a difficulty exercise.

Normally, hypotheses are formulated from observations of the researcher. From what comes in his way, the researcher forms an opinion. Due to further interest in the affair, he starts collecting data and analyses the same to draw certain conclusions. These conclusions after testing, if found verifiable, become facts and form part of the body of knowledge. In fact, the goal in observation determines the direction and stresses the facts upon which to concentrate. This finally becomes a working or exploratory hypothesis in the investigation. The explanation is viewed at the start in terms of probabilities and tentatively observed indications. Without a working hypothesis, the investigator would find the carrying of study very difficult, laborious and time consuming. The hypothesis guides him in the selection of pertinent facts needed to explain the problem at hand.

Whenever possible research should proceed from a hypothesis for without hypothesis an investigation is relatively aimless search for data of vague relevance and significance. Hypothesis is particularly necessary in the search for cause-and-effect relationship. In such cases, the presence of certain characteristics suggests correlation between variables. It gives direction to the enquiry thereby enabling the researcher to give a right focus to the study without resorting to the rule of thumb or trial and error method. It also helps the researcher to collect the specific data without wasting the time and resources. Finally, as the hypothesis is pointed and specific, appropriate and specific inferences can be drawn. As Goode and Hatt put it with out hypothesis study becomes unfocused as a random 'empirical wondering'.

Hypothesis are least crucial in studies in which the tasks determining the status of a given phenomenon, although even in such studies the investigator is likely to need some tentative hypothesis to guide him to the areas worth exploring. However, hypotheses are not essential to research, particularly in the early stages of exploration of a problem. Failure to have a hypothesis is not necessarily a sign of lack of scientific sophistication. Bacon felt that hypothesis biases the investigator towards a position and causes him to lose objectivity. This need not be so, hypothesis must be conceived as an assumption which merits consideration not as position to be defended. Furthermore, the scientific method puts such restrictions on the investigator due to the fact that he can distort evidence to fit his personal views is minimal.

Hypothesis provides direction to research and prevents the review of irrelevant literature and the collection of the data but they also ensure the collection of data necessary to answer the question posed in the statement of the problem. Hypothesis sensitises investigator to certain aspects of situation which are relevant from the standpoint of the problem at hand. In general, the hypothesis spells the difference between precision and haphazardness between fruitful and fruitless research.

Hypothesis permits the investigator to understand with greater clarity the problem and its ramification as well as the data which bear on it. They enable him to identify the procedures and methods to be used in solving his problems and rule out methods which are incapable of providing the data necessary to the hypothesis. Hypothesis also acts as a framework for the conclusions, direct answer to the hypothesis being tested.

Hypothesis can be formulated from different sources viz., experience of the researcher; from the review of literature; from the findings of the pilot study; from analysis testing the validity or otherwise of the existing theory; from the creative thinking and imagination of the researcher. As Goods and Hatt observed that general culture of the society has a great influence on the thinking process; as such hypothesis can be generated from hunch, intuition, folk wisdom, cultural patterns or metaphysical backs. Similarly, study and analysis of deviant cases also provides basis for formulating hypothesis. These are only some illustrative sources for generalizing hypothesis and by no means exhaustive. The researcher depending upon the context should identify his own sources and formulate the hypothesis.

Difficulties in the Formulation of Hypothesis

(i) Lack of acquaintance with available research.

(ii) Lack of knowledge and clarity of the theoretical framework of the area in which the investigator chooses to work.

(iii) Vagueness of the statement. For example, a course in ethics will make a student a more ethical adult.

(iv) Lack of ability to make use of the theoretical framework logically.

Need for Having a Working Hypothesis

Before one finalizes his approach to the research problem it is suggested to have a working hypothesis. It is said that such an attempt saves the investigator from becoming lost in a welter of irrelevancies. Formulation of hypothesis gives definite point to the inquiry, aids in establishing direction in which to proceed and helps to delimit the field of inquiry by singling out the pertinent fact should be set aside at least for the time being. The use of a hypothesis, thus, prevents a blind search and indiscriminate gathering of data which may later prove irrelevant to the problem under the study.

A researcher should not start out to prove the correctness of his hypotheses. He should test them and accept either negative or positive results in true scientific spirit of inquiry. In the search for truth, negative results can be just as important as positive ones. Therefore, the researcher should act like a judge which weighs the goods and bad before he can deliver a judgement.

Types of Hypotheses

Hypotheses are of different types of forms. There are hypotheses stating relationships (e.g., as cinema spreads, the crime rate increases); some specific functions null hypothesis which study the existence of no relationship between variables. Goode and Hatt have classified the hypothesis on the basis of the level of abstraction. Based on this they identified the following **three types of hypothesis:**

1. Hypothesis that states existence of empirical uniformity,
2. Those concerned with complex ideal type, and

3. Those concerned with the relation of analytic variables.

On the basis of level of abstraction, hypotheses may be classified under three categories:

The first type of hypothesis states some degree of uniformity among the empirical phenomena. For example, in an urban market like Mumbai, the determinants of demand for TV sets are identical for all the prominent makes, say, Televista, BPL, Onida, Crown, etc. It is a common sense observation.

The second type of hypothesis aims at testing the existence of logically-derived relationship between empirical uniformities. For example, we can compare, and then frame a skeptical proposition that there is some sort of relationship between the empirical uniformities:

(i) The more the entertainment programme is in colour, the more the time the viewers spend on watching the TV.

(ii) The longer the time the TV viewers view the TV programmes, the greater the demand for TVs.

The above type of relationship between the percentage of colour TV programmes and the demand for colour TVs in the city of Mumbai may be the second type of hypothesis.

The third type of hypothesis deal with a study of analytic variables between changes in one property and changes in another. The dependent variable "demand for TV" in Mumbai, Chennai and Kolkatta.

Directional Hypothesis: It states the direction or the expected outcome.

Non-directional Hypothesis: It simply states that there will be some difference between the variables, but the direction of that difference is not being predicted.

ANOVA: One statistical procedure used as a mechanism of control is analysis of covariance **(ANOVA). ANOVA** is defined as a procedure where participants' post-test scores (scores on the dependent variables obtained after the experimental treatment is given) are statistically adjusted for difference in pretest scores (pretest scores are obtained on the dependent variable before the experimental treatment is given).

Depending on the level of refinement, hypotheses are classified broadly into following two categories.

(i) Crude hypotheses; and

(ii) Refined hypotheses.

A crude hypothesis is at the low level of abstraction. It indicates the kind of data to be collected and it does not lead to higher theoretical research, in the nature of a law or a theory. The redefined type of hypothesis, on the other hand, is more significant in research and the degree of significance varies depending on the level of abstraction. Redefined hypotheses are further classified into three types:

(i) Hypotheses that state the existence of empirical uniformities.

(ii) Hypotheses that are concerned with complex ideal types.

(iii) Hypotheses that are concerned with the relation of analytical variables.

The first of hypotheses state some degree of uniformity among empirical phenomena. These hypotheses frequently though not always, represent the scientific examination of common sense propositions, for instance, as incomes of the people grow, demand for comforts also grows; similarly in urban market like Delhi, Mumbai, Chennai, and Hyderabad demand for consumer durables like refrigerators, washing machines TV sets are identical for all major brands. This is nothing but a common sense observation. There is a strong criticism that these hypotheses do not serve as useful ones, particularly in social research.

The second type of refined hypothesis aims at testing the existence of logically derived relationship between empirical uniformities. For example, we may propose the following sort of relationship between empirical uniformities in relation to the demand for colour TVs in a city like Hyderabad.

(i) There exist a high relation between the demand for colour TVs and colour programmes televised;

(ii) The more the sponsored programmes in TV the higher the demand for TV sets;

(iii) The more the number of salary revisions and bonus payments, the more is the demand for V sets; and

(iv) The lower the difference between the cost of black and white and Colour TVs, the higher is the demand for Colour TVs.

Likewise, we can develop various types of relationship and then test for acceptance or rejection.

The third type of hypothesis occurs at a level of abstraction beyond that of ideal types. They deal with a study of analytical variables between changes in one property and changes in another. To continue our example, the sort of relationship that prevails under this category would be between the demand for TV sets (dependent variable) and various other factors (independent variables) like other modes of entertainment available, the incomes of the inhabitants, the demonstration effect, the advertisement impact created by the TV companies and the general broadcasting policy of the Government. Therefore, the demand for a particular brand model or range of TV sets can be studied in relation to many of these variables and the change in the independent variables can be hypothesized and tested with the help of statistical methods.

NULL HYPOTHESES

Besides the above, there is a mention of null hypothesis in research. This is a statistical proposition invented by Sir Ronald Fisher. It essentially states that there is no relation between the variables of concerned. For example, there is no significant difference in the instructional standard of single shift and double shift industries. Commenting on the use of null hypothesis Prof. Kerlinger opined that this is a poor practice because it begs the scientific question. To take an example instead of saying that method 'A' is more conductive to learning arithmetic than method 'B', the researcher may say that there is no difference between methods A and B, though the investigator believes that method A is superior to method B. The hypothesis is MA = MB. The result would be MA > MB or MA < MB. In this process, the power of substantive hypothesis is lost.

In its sample form the null hypothesis asserts that there is no relationship or dependence between the two variables that are sought to be related. The null hypothesis is akin to the legal principle that a man is innocent until he is proved guilty. It constituted a challenge. The function of the experiment, observation or analysis of data is to give the facts a chance to refuse or fail to refute this challenge. Thus, when we want to relate educational attainments and profits earned by businessmen, the first hypothesis we formulate is the null hypothesis. Ho, states that there is no relationship between educational attainments and profits. The alternate hypothesis, Ha, naturally would be that educational attainments and profits are related. But in practice these two hypotheses may not be stated but would be kept in view by the researcher. Depending upon the outcome of computations, either of these two hypotheses will be accepted and the fact will then be stated.

However, these hypotheses are frequently used, in subjects like mathematics, statistics. In fact, the Nobel Prize winners in economics, Modigiani and Miller have used this type of a hypotheses in one of their theories on dividend policy.

Declarative Form: It generally states a relationship between the variables concerned. For example, we can state that there will be a significant difference in the instructional standards for boys and girls schools.

Prediction Form: It is chosen because it allows the research worker to state principles which he actually expects to emerge from the experiment. This type of hypothesis is more useful in action research studies.

Question Form: The Declarative form of hypothesis in question form may read– "Is there a significant difference in the instructional standards of boys and girls schools?".

The Functions of Hypothesis

It is indicated in the earlier discussion that hypothesis is a logical starting point in the search for the facts or truth. In this sense, the chief function of hypothesis is to provide a useful direction to the researcher. It serves as a basis for his future endeavour. Unless a researcher knows what he wants to verify or test, the search becomes unguided. That is why hypothesis is said to be proposition which can be put to a test to determine its validity. The proposition may prove to be correct or incorrect; but it leads one to an empirical test.

The second function of the hypothesis is that it serves as a basis for future knowledge. A hypothesis after verification and testing emerges as a sound body of knowledge. When facts are drawn, they constitute a theory. As such, the relation between theory and hypothesis is very close. As William H. George has observed, "In practice a theory is an elaborate hypothesis which deals with more types of facts than does the simple hypothesis". In the words of Goode and Hatt every worthwhile theory permits the formulation of additional hypotheses. These when tested are either proved or disproved and in turn constitute further tests of the original theory.

Another purpose of the hypothesis is its utility in explaining the social phenomenon. When hypotheses are tested, they explain the social phenomenon associated with them. The phenomena may be totally new or partly known or not known earlier.

Characteristics of a Good and Usable Hypothesis

If a hypothesis is required to serve the purpose for which it is intended, it should have certain basic characteristics. These characteristics are aptly described by William J. Goode and Paul K. Hatt in their methods in social research. Let us briefly discuss some of these characteristics.

1. ***Conceptual Clarity:*** The hypothesis to be framed must be conceptually clear. As far as possible care must be taken to definite the terms used in the formulation in precise language.
2. ***Empirical Reference:*** If hypothesis is to be useful, it should contain only such propositions which are verifiable or suitable for empirical analysis.
3. ***Specific in Nature:*** The hypothesis must be formulated in specific terms. There should be no room for ambiguity.
4. ***Related to Available Techniques:*** An investigation to be practical should relate the hypotheses to the investigational techniques feasible in the par-

ticular science. This requires the researcher to have a sound knowledge of techniques to test the hypothesis and thus to formulate practical questions. If on the other hand, in can never be tested.

5. ***Related to a Body of Theory:*** Many a time investigators would be swayed away by their fascination to the things, without bothering much whether the inquiry will help to refuse or support the existing theoretical base. As such the work taken up by the researcher must be related to a body of theory.

PROBLEMS IN FORMULATION OF HYPOTHESIS

If hypothesis is to serve as an effective guide for future inquiry, it must be formulated with due care.

Absence of Theoretical Base: If hypothesis is to be proved effective, it must be related to a body of theory. Unfortunately, the investigator may not find such a base existing several times. The question then would be what to do? The duty of the researcher is to go on formulating his own propositions, so long as they are found reasonable and appealing to the common sense at least.

Lack of Ability to Use the Framework Logically: Not only that the propositions formulated need to have relation to the theory, but also they must be used to the correct sense in a logical manner.

Failure to Acquaint with Techniques: The other problem with the formulation of hypothesis is the failure of the researcher to acquaint with the techniques used to test the hypothesis. Lack of knowledge in this area leads to imprecise and meaningless formulation of proposition.

SOURCE OF HYPOTHESES

Hypothesis can be formulated from different sources viz., personal experience and intimate knowledge of the facts of the real world, experience of the researcher from the review of literature, from the findings of the pilot study, from analysis, testing or otherwise of the existing theory, from the creative thinking and imagination of the researcher. Deep erudition and mastery of the theory and literature is a necessary condition for formulation of hypothesis. Positive statements in economics are a source of hypothesis. They explain 'what is' and not 'what ought to be.'

Analogy from other sciences: Economics has borrowed many an expression from physics. For example, coefficient of expansion of demand (heat in physics).

Fiction: The social novel brings to the reader the various social forces at work.

As such hypothesis can be generated from hunch intuition, folk wisdom cultural patterns etc.

(i) A hypothesis arises from intuition.

(ii) A hypothesis also arises from other studies. The findings of a study may be formulated as hypothesis.

(iii) Theory is the seed bed of hypothesis.

(iv) Personal happiness provides scope for hypothesis. Happiness has been correlated with income, education, occupation, social class and so on.

Criteria for Judging Hypothesis

Merit of a hypothesis can be judged only by its effectiveness. Nevertheless we can set general criteria for judging the effectiveness of hypothesis.

A good hypothesis must be based directly on existing data. It might even be expected to predict or anticipate previously unknown data. It must explain existing data in simpler terms and as concisely as possible. A good hypothesis must above all be testable.

Goode and Hatt suggest the following characteristics of a useful hypothesis:

1. Must be conceptually clear;
2. Should have empirical reference;
3. Must be specific;
4. Should be related to available techniques; and
5. Should be related to a body of theory.

Some assert that hypothesis may be stated as a question though there is no general consensus on this view. It can be stated in a question form or in the form a declaration of statement or in the form of a directional statement or in a null form.

There are several problems in formulating the hypothesis. The chief difficulties according to Goode and Hatt are:

1. Absence of a clear theoretical framework;
2. Lack of ability to utilize that theoretical framework logically; and
3. Failure to be acquainted with available research techniques so as to be able to phrase the hypothesis properly.

After the formulation of hypothesis, the researcher should collect the data by choosing the appropriate tools and analyze the data based on the requirements. The data so collected, may support the hypothesis or disprove the hypothesis.

The formulation of problem, thus, involves several steps like choosing the broad area of the research, identifying the research problem within the broad area and finally formulation of a hypothesis.

IMPORTANCE OF HYPOTHESIS

Whenever possible research should proceed from a hypothesis, Without hypothesis an investigation is relatively aimless search. Hypothesis is particularly necessary in the search for cause and effect relationship. The presence of certain characteristics does suggest correlation between variables. It gives direction to the enquiry thereby enabling the researcher to give a right focus to the study without resorting to rule of thumb or trial and error method. It also helps the researcher to collect the specific data without wasting the line and resources. Finally, as the hypothesis is specific, appropriate and specific inferences can be drawn.

Hypothesis provides direction to research and prevents the review of irrelevant literature and the collection of useless or excess data. Hypothesis not only prevents waste in the collection of data, but they also ensure the collection of data necessary to answer the question posed in the statement of the problem.

UTILITY OF HYPOTHESIS

The utility of hypothesis for social research may be summed up under the following heads.

(a) **Hypothesis provides guidance to proceed on certain definite lines:** Hypothesis helps the investigator in knowing the direction in which he should proceed. In the absence of hypothesis the researcher is like a sailor on an unchartered vessel without compass or rudder.

To consider specifically the role of hypothesis in determining the direction of research, we might turn again to the hypothesis concerning husbands and wives and their perceptions of their respective role in consumer decision making. The hypothesis specifies who shall be studied, in what context they shall be studied (their consumer decision making) and what shall be studied (their individual perceptions of their roles in the purchase or consumer decision making situations). The study should clearly, therefore, not involve itself in seeking information about other types of roles which husband and wife might play. Another suggestions that might flow from a reflection upon this hypothesis is that we might find that husbands and wives to disagree on their perceptions of roles but these differences may be explained in terms of additional variables such as age, social class, background; personality differences, and other factors not associated with their differences of sex.

(b) **Hypothesis helps in selecting pertinent factors:** Pauline Y. Young has rightly remarked. The use of hypothesis prevents a blind search and indiscriminate gathering of masses of data which may later prove irrelevant to the problem under study.

(c) **Hypothesis helps in drawing specific conclusions:** If hypothesis is rightly drawn and scientifically formulated, it helps the researcher not only to proceed in this study on right lines but also to draw conclusions. Goode and Hatt have aptly said :

"Without hypothesis the research is unfocussed as a random empirical wandering. The results cannot be stated/studied as facts with clear meaning. Hypothesis is a necessary link between theory and investigations, which lead to discovery of additional to knowledge".

Thus hypothesis is the integral part of scientific research and without the former the latter shall neither be valuable nor possible. To sum up, hypothesis is the foundation of scientific social research.

(d) A tentative solution posed on a cursory observation of known and available data and adopted provisionally to explain certain events and to guide in the investigation of others. It is, in fact, a possible solution to the problems. (M.H. Gopal).

TESTING OF HYPOTHESIS

There are two important means of testing hypothesis:

(i) The study of hypothesis for logical consistency, and

(ii) The study of hypothesis for agreement with fact.

A hypothesis is never proved, it is merely sustained or rejected. The hypotheses that are formulated need to be tested for their acceptance or rejection. In fact, only those hypotheses that are suitably tested for their significance are to be studied form part of the body of knowledge. Normally the hypothesis is tested by making use of a predefined decision rule, which is applied to sample data and which guides the researcher in deciding whether to accept or reject the hypothesis on the basis of the outcome of the sample or samples drawn. There are two fairly important means of testing hypothesis: (i) the study of hypothesis for logical consistency; and (ii) the study of hypothesis for agreement with fact.

(i) The study of hypothesis for logical consistency is a phase of thinking. It consists of checking the logical characters of the reasoning by which the consequences of hypotheses are deducted for verification. In the second place the study of hypothesis for logical consistency involves checking it for agreement with the already known laws of nature it must not conflict the highest and simplest laws of good thinking and it must not disagree with those principles of science which are considered valid beyond reasonable doubt. The suggested inferences are tested in though, for logical coherence before they are tested in action. For instance, Modigliani and Miller's hypothesis regarding capital structure falls in this category. They have hypothesised that:

(ii) Given the assumptions M and M argue that for firms in the same risk class the total market value is independent of the debt-equity ratio and is given by capitalizing the expected net operating income by the rate appropriate to that risk class. This is expressed by them as follows:

$$V = S + D = X/K_0 \ \frac{NI}{K_0}$$

where V = market value of the firm

S = market value of equity

D = market value of debt

X = the expected net operating income

K_0 = the capitalization rate appropriate to the risk class of the firm.

(iii) For any firm in a given risk, the cost of equity capital K_e is equal to the constant average cost of capital K_0, plus a premium for the financial risk. Which is equal to debt-equity ratio spread between the constant average cost of capital and the cost of debt:

Thus $K_e = K_0 + (K_0 - K_d)/D/S$

where K_e = cost of equity capital

K_0 = constant average cost of capital

K_d = cost of debt capital

D/S = debt equity ratio.

These propositions were tested by Modigliani and Millar for their logical consistency and they could prove their hypothesis with the help of 'Arbitrage Process'.

A well known example of the test of hypothesis in the realm of management science is in the area of statistical quality control. Tests have been reduced to standardized procedures that enable the management to discover variation in the quality of production or the quality of goods supplied by the suppliers. It facilitates the determination of an acceptable quality level for all incoming lots.

In the study of hypothesis for agreement with facts, one argues whether the hypothesis is true or false under the given conditions. Then one probes into whether these conditions are present. If these conditions are not present, then he should restate his hypothesis and collect fresh evidence for making the study worthwhile. After testing a hypothesis it may be accepted or rejected. Sometimes, the facts and data may suggest revision or modification of the hypothesis.

For the purpose of testing the hypothesis one may have to resort to various types of techniques to test and analyze both quantitative and qualitative factors involved. Various statistical, mathematical, econometric and experimental methods are now available to test different kinds of hypotheses. The hope that a common procedure would be suitable for testing any hypothesis is a distant possibility. The technique to be adopted depends upon convenience, availability and reliability of data, knowledge of the researcher and finally the level of sophistification required. A brief description and utility of the various techniques available for testing hypothesis is provided separately in this book.

There are two approaches to hypothesis testing – sampling theory approach and Bayesian approach.

The sampling theory approach (traditional approach) is found in all Statistics Books. It is widely used in research. The decision making rests upon the sampling data.

The Bayesian approach is an extension of the classical approach, which use sampling data for making decision. It also incorporates all other information available to the decision makers. Most of the additional information consists of subjective probability estimates.

Collection of data is an important requirement in the testing of hypothesis. Details regarding what data and how it should be collected must be decided upon in the light of operational definitions which are precisely and specifically defined. For example, when we try to relate educational attainments, it can have various references, whether we should take those who have just passes certain examinations or those who just studied in certain classes or courses. What we regards as higher educational attainments must be defined. An operational definition can be that those who have secured a degree of any university or any higher qualification may be regarded as having higher educational attainments and those who did not secure the degree including those who joined a degree programme but could not complete and pass the examination would have to be regarded as having lower academic attainments. It we define higher educational attainments in another way, the ranks secured by the businessman when they studied can also be used. But this may not be as feasible and objective as the requirement of the degree in the earlier case since awarding of ranks may not be the practice in many schools and since ranks may not be objectively reported.

Then it is possible to demarcate the various levels of educational attainments within certain limits – class intervals like no education, 1st to V standard, V to VIII standard, VIII to HSLC, degree etc. and clearly define the class intervals stating what are included and what are excluded. In fact educational attainments can be operationally defined in several ways.

Just as we define educational attainments, profits can also be defined and put into various brackets or class intervals.

Once the detailed information pertaining to both these variables are collected in terms of operational references, it is possible to present data pertaining to one against the data pertaining to the other and then interpret. The outcome it may come out is that an over-whelming number of these with more educational attainments did earn more profit in which case, we can say that the hypothesis is true. But in many situations variables like these do not present truly convincing results to enable the researcher to come to clear conclusions.

It is probable that some of the less educated respondents could earn more profits – may be due to their long experience (an intervening variable which did not separate) or may be due to reason that more educated people hesitate to bribe officials to permit them resort to unfair means of trade like evasion of taxes, unrecorded turnover etc. It may also happen that the business ethics of the less educated are favorable for earning more profits. Due to these or other reasons, when we put profits against educational attainments, the pattern which emerges may not help us to arrive a simple decision.

In the case of business research involving a hypothesis where historical data is to be used, collecting and presenting such relevant objective data from authentic primary and secondary sources will establish the hypothesis. More authentic and strong the evidence, more sound and reliable will be the conclusion. Use of statistical techniques will be ruled out in many of the cases although they may become operational in some contexts where a series of information or data that could be tabulated is available.

In the case of hypothesis involving experimental design of research, the experiment will have to be performed to verify the hypothesis. For example, the hypothesis that coffee taken in the night makes a man sleepless can be tested by giving coffee several times to a number of persons and then observing their sleeping pattern; if all of them experience sleeplessness we draw the inference that the hypothesis is proved. There will be some difficulty that some people get sleep and some others do not. It is in this situation quantitative techniques are to be used. In the simplest case we took at the percentage of people who had sleep and compare it with those who were sleepless. Now a decision can be taken based on these percentages. If some rigorous testing is required, the quantity of coffee and the time of sleep or sleeplessness can be correlated by means of correlation analysis. Many tests of significance of relation between these two can be made use of. But in the case of such a simple experiment, there are many intervening variables like the prior sleeping habits, coffee drinking habits, health conditions etc., of the persons subjected to the experiment which also will influence the length of sleep. If we want higher degree of abstraction it becomes necessary to eliminate the influence of all the interviewing variables. Even the vary knowledge that these respondents are being subjected to an experiment will push them to a different motivational stage interfering their sleeping pattern. This point was an unexpected finding in Hawthorne experiments.

HYPOTHESIS TESTING PROCEDURE

The first step in testing the hypothesis is setting up of hypothesis. The conventional approach is to set up two hypotheses instead of one. If one hypothesis is true, the other is false. Alternatively if one hypothesis is rejected then the other is accepted. These hypotheses are (i) Null hypotheses and (ii) alternative hypotheses.

The second step in choosing a statistical technique: There are many statistical tests, which are frequently used in hypothesis testing. They are "z" test, "t" test, "F" test and chi-square test. The researcher should be able to choose the appropriate test.

The third step is the selection of desired level of significance. The confidence with which the experiment rejects or retains a hypothesis depends upon the level expressed in percentage such as 5%, 1% LOS (Level of significance) etc.

The final step in hypothesis is to draw statistical decision involving the acceptance or rejection of hypothesis. This will defend on whether the computed value of the test falls in the region of acceptance or in the region of rejection at a given level of significance.

HYPOTHESES TESTED

1. Large firms with richer resources are more multi product firms.
2. The firms which diversify their productive base are likely to grow faster than those whose output remain homogeneous.
3. Older firms are more prone to adopt diversification strategies than younger ones.
4. Firms with an unsatisfactory profit and cost record are likely to diversify more.

Statistical Inference

It is high fashion to try the use of statistical inference for almost anything and everything these days in decision situations. Many researchers also have become victims of this mania although many business and behavioural situations can not be subjected to strict statistical abstraction.

Statistical techniques are used for testing the direction and strength of the relations once the variables are related. Statistical inference refers the process of selecting and using a sample data to draw inference about a population based on a subject of it – namely the sample drawn from the population.

The procedure for testing a hypothesis and drawing inference with statistical significance levels may be described as follows:

FORMULATE HYPOTHESIS

Although we say we test a hypothesis, it is custom to formulate hypotheses even though these are not specifically written down. These hypothesis must be constructed in such a manner that if one hypothesis is rejected the other is accepted and vice-versa. The two hypotheses are known as

(i) Null hypothesis and

(ii) Alternative hypothesis.

Significance Level

Having formulated the hypothesis the next step would be to test the validity of Ho (null hypothesis) against Ha (alternate hypothesis) at a certain level of significance. Acceptance or rejection of the hypothesis would depend upon the significance level adopted. Significance level is customarily expressed as a percentage say 5%, 1% etc. A level of significance of say 5% would mean that the probability of rejecting a true hypothesis is 5%. In other words in 5% of the cases the decision arrived at may go wrong, i.e., the decision will be true in 95% of the cases. By testing it at 1% level of significance this risk is further reduced. The stratification can now say that in 99% of the cases a true hypothesis will not be rejected and in 1% of cases a true hypothesis may be rejected.

Setting a Test Criterion

The next step will be to determine the test criterion to be used if a very direct and linear relationship is anticipated between the two variables. Correlation and regression analysis can be chosen. But in very many situations in business research the variable may not have very strong relations mainly because of their non-parametric characteristics and the indirect involvement of many intervening variables which could be very difficult to eliminate. Thus we have to choose only the probability distribution that can be applied to the sample data. Some of these distributions are t, F and χ^2. Test criteria must employ an appropriate probability distribution; for example, if only a small sample is available, the use of normal distribution will not be appropriate, while "t" distribution might serve the purpose.

When it is not possible to make a rigid assumption about the distribution of the population from which samples are being drawn, we have to make use of non-parametric or distribution free method chi-square test of independence and goodness of fit is a paramount examples of the use of non-parametric tests.

It is not possible to describe exhaustively all the statistical tests that are used in hypothesis testing. Let us discuss only one test that is chi-square test.

CHI-SQUARE TEST

The chi-square test is one of the simplest and most widely used non-parametric tests in statistical work. The Greek letter χ^2 was first used by Karl Pearson in the year 1900. The quantity χ^2 describes the magnitude of the discrepancy between theory and observation. It is defined as:

$$\chi^2 = \frac{\Sigma(O - E)^2}{E}$$

where O = Observed frequency.

Σ = Sum of the differences between observed and expected frequencies E refers to the expected frequencies.

The observed frequencies are those collected or observed. The expected frequencies are the theoretical frequencies.

The above formula is used in the following manner:

(i) First, expected frequencies are calculated.

(ii) Secondly, after getting the difference between observed and expected frequencies (O-E), the differences are squared.

(iii) The figures obtained in step (ii) are divided by expected frequencies.

(iv) The summation of items obtained in step (iii) gives the value of Chi-square.

Expected frequencies can be found by the formula

$$E = \frac{RT \times CT}{N}$$

where RT = Row total, CT = Column total

and N = total number of observations.

The Chi-square test is widely used as a non-parametric test in statistical work. With the help of Chi-square test we are in a position to know whether a given difference between actual and expectation has been caused by a chance or whether it has resulted in because of the inadequacy of the theory to fit the observed facts.

The steps in computing χ^2 are the following:

(i) Preparation of Contingency Table

It is presumed that all the steps laid down in earlier sections pertaining to the formulation of hypothesis and definition concepts in terms of empirical references are gone through. If the whole universe cannot be enumerated, selection of an appropriate sample becomes necessary. Using the data collection tools, required data is also collected. The data pertaining to the variables that are to be related are now presented as a contingency table which by itself will be enabling some inference. It is only because we want higher levels of abstraction, we subject this table for further treatment. Assume that the data collected are presented in the Table below.

Table 5.1: Level of Education of Businessmen and the Net Profits Earned by Them

Level of Education	Net up to 50	Profit 50-100	Earned in Rs. 000 Above 100	Total
Below SSLC	8	6	6	20
SSLC and Hr. Sec.	18	7	5	30
Degree and Above	30	10	10	50
Total	56	23	21	100

(ii) Calculation of Expected Frequencies

Using the formula for expected frequency, $E = \frac{RT \times CT}{N}$, calculate expected values for all frequencies. If any cell frequency is zero, the table will have to be edited by merging one column of row with another so that some cell value other than 0 is obtained. If the degree of freedom is 1, then it is important to see that the expected cell frequency is at least 5, although 10 will be better. For degree of freedom exceeding say 3 to 4 and N very large, this condition is not important since the distribution would tend to become normal. But even in such cases it is necessary to eliminate zero from cell frequencies by combining those rows or columns with other appropriately. This is because existence of zeros will make χ^2 zero.

(iii) Determining Degree of Freedom

Degree of freedom is calculated by the formula (R – 1) (C – 1), where R = Number of rows and C = Number of columns. When there are more rows and columns, naturally the degrees of freedom also will become larger indicating that the total number of observations, N is also larger. Results of χ^2 test will be more reliable when degrees of freedom and N are larger. In the Table 5.1, the degree of freedom is 4 because there are 3 rows and 3 columns and D.F. = (3 – 1) (3 – 1) = 2 × 2 = 4.

(iv) *Other Calculations*

Table 5.2 represents the other calculations. For the first observed cell value of 8, the expected frequency is calculated by taking the formula = $\frac{RT \times CT}{N}$.

Applying this we get $\frac{20 \times 56}{100} = 11.2$

Similarly for the next cell value in the same column namely 18, it is $\frac{30 \times 56}{100}$ = 16.8, that way expected frequencies are calculated for all cell values and these appear under column E, in the next column we write down the difference between observed and expected values. Signs are not important here since we square the differences in the next column. The squared values of the earlier columns are divided by E. The sum total of this column gives the calculated χ^2 of the observed values.

Calculation of χ^2; Using Data from Table:

Table 5.2

O	E	O – E	$(O - E)^2/E$
8	11.2	3.2	0.9143
18	16.8	1.2	0.0857
30	28.0	2.0	0.1429
6	4.6	1.4	0.4261
7	6.9	0.1	0.0014
10	11.5	1.5	0.1957
6	4.2	1.8	0.7714
5	6.3	1.3	0.2683
10	10.5	0.5	0.0230
			2.82941

[Degree of freedom = (R – 1) (C – 1) = (3 – 1) (3 – 1) = 4. For D.F. 4, the χ^2 table value at 5% level of significance = 9.488. The calculated χ^2 = 2.8294 which is mush smaller than the table value.]

(v) *Comparison of Observed with the Theoretical Value*

Inference is arrived at by making comparison of the calculated χ^2 with the relevant table value. Statistical tables with χ^2 values for different degrees of freedom at different levels of significance are available. One has to consult those tables. For example, the calculated χ^2 in our example is 2.829. The degree of freedom was 4. If the desired level of significance is 5% the table value χ^2 is 9.488 for 4 degrees of freedom. (The calculated χ^2 = 2.829 and the table value = 9.488). Since the table value is higher and the calculated value lower, the inference would be that there is no association between the two attributes namely educational attainments and profits earned by businessman. In this context we have evidence only to confirm the null hypothesis that there is no relationship between level of education of businessmen and the net profits earned by them. Thus, in this case there is no need to adopt the alternate hypothesis and we confirm the null hypothesis.

On the other hand consider that the data we obtained from the filled or from secondary source concerning these two variables are in the given below:

Level of Educational of Businessman and the net profits earned by them, Net profit earned in Rs. 000

Level of Education	up to 50	50 – 100	Above 100	Total
Below SSLC	8	5	9	22
SSLC and Hr. Sec.	10	15	9	34
Degree and above	8	10	26	44
Total	26	30	44	100

The chi-square has been calculated as follows:

Table 5.3: Calculation of Chi-square Test

O	E	O – E	$(O - E)^2$	$(O - E)^2/E$
8	5.72	2.28	5.1984	0.9088
10	8.84	1.16	1.3456	0.1522
8	11.44	3.44	11.8336	1.0344
5	6.60	1.60	2.5600	C.3879
15	10.20	4.80	23.0400	2.2588
10	13.20	3.20	10.2400	0.7758
9	9.68	0.68	0.4624	0.0478
9	14.96	5.96	35.5216	2.3744
26	19.36	6.64	44.0896	2.2744
			Total	10.2173

Calculated value of χ^2 = 10.2173

D.F = 4; Table value = 9.488

Since the table value is less than the Calculated value of χ^2 we reject the null hypothesis.

Hence, the alternate hypothesis that there is relationship between educational attainment and net profits of businessmen is accepted. On looking at the table it is evident 'the higher the educational attainments more will be the profits'.

THE 't' TEST

Sir William Gosset developed a significance test and through it made a significant contribution in the theory of sampling applicable in case of small samples. The test is commonly known as student 't' test and is based on the 't' contribution in which the statistic 't' is defined as

$$t = \frac{\bar{x}\mu}{s} \times \sqrt{n}$$

where $\bar{x}$ = mean of the sample

μ = mean of the population

n = number of items in the sample

$$s = \sqrt{\frac{\Sigma(x - \bar{x})^2}{n - 1}}$$

For applying this test in context of small samples, the 't' value is calculated first of all and then is compared with table value of 't' at certain level of significance for given degrees of freedom. If the calculated value of 't' exceeds the tabulated value (say 't' 0.05) we infer that the difference is significant at 5% level but if 't' is less than the concerned table value of the 't', the difference is not treated as significant.

A Note on the t-table

The body of the 't' table provides the 't' value corresponding to a degree of freedom and tail area. Therefore, to use the t-table we need to know the two numbers–the tail area and the numbers. For one tail test at 5% level of significance the table value is denoted by t. 05v. On the other hand if a two tail test is performed at the same 5% level of significance, the table value is denoted by t.025v in the first case. The tail area in the first case is 0.5 where as in the second case it is half of it viz., .025

APPLICATIONS OF 't' TEST

(1) To test the significance of the mean of a random sample

$$t = \frac{|\bar{x} - \mu|}{\sqrt{\frac{\Sigma(x - \bar{x})^2}{n - 1}}} \sqrt{n}$$

Illustration

Ten specimens of copper wires drawn from a large lot have the following breaking strength (in kg. wt.):

578, 572, 570, 568, 572, 578, 570, 572, 596, 544

Test whether the mean breaking strength of the lot may be taken to be 578 kg. wt.

Solution:

We take the hypothesis that there is no difference between the mean strength of the universe and that of the lot. Then on the basis of the sample data, the mean and standard deviation have been worked out as under:

Table 5.4: Mean and Standard Deviation

x	$(x - \bar{x})$	$(x - \bar{x})^2$
578	6	36
572	0	0
570	– 2	4
568	– 4	16
572	0	0
578	6	36
570	– 2	4
572	0	0
596	24	576
544	– 28	784
5720		1456

$$\bar{x} = \frac{\Sigma x}{n} = \frac{5720}{10} = 572 \text{ (mean)}$$

$$s = \frac{\sqrt{\Sigma(x - \bar{x})^2}}{n - 1} = \frac{\sqrt{1456}}{10 - 1} = \frac{\sqrt{1456}}{9} = 12.72$$

$$t = \frac{|\overline{x} - \mu|}{S} = \sqrt{n}$$

$$= \frac{|572-578|}{12.72} \times \sqrt{10} = \frac{6}{12.72} = 3.162$$

$$= \frac{18.972}{12.72} = 1.49$$

Degrees of freedom n – 1 = 9

At 5% level of significance for 9 d.f. the table value of t = 2.262.

The calculated value, of t is less than the table value. Hence the difference is in significant. The mean breaking strength of the lot may be 578 kg. wt. with 95% confidence level.

(2) To test the difference between the mean of two samples

$$t = \frac{\overline{x}_1 - \overline{x}_2}{\sqrt{\frac{\Sigma(x_1 - x_1)^2 + (x_2 - \overline{x})^2}{n_1 + n_2 - 2}}\sqrt{\frac{1}{n_1} + \frac{1}{n_2}}}$$

Illustration

Sample of sales in similar shops in two towns all taken for a new product with the following results.

	Mean sales	*Variance*	*Size of sample*
Town A	*57*	*5.3*	*5*
Town B	*61*	*4.8*	*7*

Is there any evidence of difference in sales in the two towns?

Solution

We take the hypothesis that there is no difference between the two sample means concerning states in the two towns. Then we workout 't' value as follows:

$$t = \frac{\overline{x}_1 - \overline{x}_2}{\sqrt{\frac{\Sigma(x_1 - x_1)^2 + (x_2 - \overline{x})^2}{n_1 + n_2 - 2}}\sqrt{\frac{1}{n_1} + \frac{1}{n_2}}}$$

For town A

variance $= \frac{\Sigma(x_1 - \overline{x}_1)^2}{n_1} = 5.3 = \frac{\Sigma(x_1 - \overline{x}_1)^2}{5} = 5.3$

$\therefore \quad \Sigma(x_1 - \overline{x}_1)^2 = 5.3 \times 5 = 26.5$

For town B

$$\text{variance} = \frac{\Sigma(x_2 - \bar{x}_2)^2}{n_2}$$

$$= \frac{\Sigma(x_2 - \bar{x}_2)^2}{7} = 4.8$$

$$\therefore \quad \Sigma(x_2 - x_2)^2 = 4.8^k\ 7 = 33.6$$

$$\therefore \quad t = \frac{\bar{x}_1 - \bar{x}_2}{\sqrt{\dfrac{\Sigma(x_1 - x_1)^2 + \Sigma(x_2 - \bar{x})^2}{n_1 + n_2 - 2}}\sqrt{\dfrac{1}{n_1} \times \dfrac{1}{n_2}}}$$

$$= \frac{|57 - 61|}{\dfrac{\sqrt{26.5 + 33.6}}{5 + 7 - 2}} = \sqrt{\frac{1}{5} + \frac{1}{7}}$$

$$= \frac{4}{\dfrac{\sqrt{60.1}}{10}\ \dfrac{\sqrt{7 + 5}}{35}}$$

$$= \frac{4}{2.4}\ 5.8 = \frac{4}{1.421}$$

$$t = 2.82$$

Degrees of freedom = $n_1 + n_2 - 2 - 6 = +7 = 10$

Table value of t at 5% level of significance for 10 d.f. is 2.228.

∴ The calculated value of t is greater than its table value. Hence the hypothesis is rejected and the difference is significant.

(3) To test significance of an observed correlation coefficient

$$t = \frac{r}{\sqrt{(1 - r)^2}} \times \sqrt{n - 2}$$

Illustration

It was found that the coefficient of correlation between two variables calculated from a sample of 26 items was 0.37. Test the significance of r at 5% level with the help of t test.

Solution

$$t = \frac{r}{\sqrt{(1 - r)^2}} \times \sqrt{n - 2}$$

$$= \frac{0.37}{\sqrt{1 - (.37)^2}} \times \sqrt{25 - 2}$$

$$= \frac{3.37}{\sqrt{1-0.1369}} \times \sqrt{23}$$

$$= \frac{0.37 \times 4.796}{0.93} = 1.093$$

Degrees of freedom n – 2 = 25 – 2 = 23. The table value of t at 5% level of significant for 23 d.f. = 2. 059.

The calculated value of t is less than table value of t. Hence r is not significant.

(4) Difference test

This is used in the context of paired data.

$$t = \frac{\text{Meanofdifference}}{\text{S.D. of difference}} \times \sqrt{n}$$

Illustration

The sales data of an item in six shops before and after a special promotional campaign are:

Shops	A	B	C	D	E	F
Before the campaign	58	28	31	48	50	42
After the campaign	58	29	30	55	56	45

Can the campaign be judged to be a success? Test at 5% level of significance.

Solution

We take the hypothesis that the campaign does not bring any improvement in sales. In order to judge this we apply the difference test. For this purpose, we calculate the mean and S.D. of the difference in two sample items as follows:

Shops	Sales before campaign	Sales after campaign	Difference	(D – D)	$(D - D)^2$
A	53	58	5	1.5	2.25
B	28	29	1	– 2.5	6.25
C	31	30	– 1	– 4.5	20.25
D	48	55	7	3.5	12.25
E	50	56	6	2.5	6.25
F	42	45	3	– 0.5	0.25
	Total		21		47.50

$$\text{Mean of difference} = -\frac{\Sigma D}{n}\Sigma = -\frac{21}{6} = 3.5$$

$$\text{S.D. of difference} = \sqrt{\frac{\Sigma(D-D)^2}{n-1}} = \sqrt{\frac{47.50}{6-1}}$$

$$= \sqrt{\frac{47.5}{5}} = \sqrt{9.5} = 3.08$$

$$t = \frac{\text{Mean of difference}}{\text{S.D. of difference}} \times \sqrt{n}$$

$$= \frac{3.5}{3.08} \times \sqrt{6} = 1.14 \times 2.45 = 2.793$$

Degree of freedom 6 – 1 = 5.

The table value of t at 5% level of significance for 5 d.f. = 2.571.

Since the calculated value of t is greater than its table value, the difference is significant. Thus, the hypothesis is rejected and the special promotional campaign can be taken as a success.

F-TEST

F-test is generally known as variance ratio test and is mostly used in context of analysis of variance. In context of sampling the object of this test is to test the hypothesis whether the two samples are from same normal population with equal variance. The statistic F is calculated as under.

$$F = \frac{\sigma_1^2}{\sigma_2^2}$$

where

$$\sigma_1^2 = \frac{\Sigma(x_1 - \bar{x}_1)^2}{(n_1 - x_1)}$$

$$\sigma_2^2 = \frac{\Sigma(x_2 - \bar{x}_2)^2}{(n_2 - 1)}$$

σ_1^2 is treated greater than σ_2^2, which means that the numerator is always the greater. Variance tables have been prepared by statisticians for the variance ratio F at different levels of significance. By comparing the observed values of F with the table values we can conclude whether the difference between the samples could have arisen due to chance fluctuations. If the values of F is greater than F 0.05 for $(n_1 - 1)$ and $(n_2 - 1)$. We regard the ratio as significant at 5% level. Degrees of freedom for greater variance is represented as V and degrees of freedom, for smaller variance as v. On the other hand, if F is less than F 0.05 we shall conclude that samples could have come from two normal population with the same variance or from two normal populations. The following example will illustrate the application of F test.

Illustration

Central Cereal Ltd., a manufacturer of chemical funnel, found that batch to batch variability of recovery was too high. The firm then made certain adjustments in the control panel of the distillation column hoping to reduce the variability of recovery percentage. Two samples were taken, one before the adjustment and the other after the adjustment. The observed sample data regarding percentage recovery of funnel were as follows.

Sample 1 (Before adjustment): 1.1, 1.4, 1.7, 3.2, 3.6, 4.6, 5.4

Sample 2 (After adjustment): 1.2, 1.5, 2.1, 2.4, 2.6, 3.1, 3.4, 4.2, 5.6.

Does this provide sufficient evidence to conclude that the necessary percentage has changed after adjustment?

Solution

Taking the hypothesis that the two samples are drawn from the same normal population we solve the question as under.

Sample I			Sample II		
x_1	$(x_1 - \bar{x}_1)$	$(x_1 - \bar{x}_1)^2$	x_2	$(x_2 - \bar{x}_2)$	$(x_2 - \bar{x}_2)^2$
1.1	– 1.9	3.61	1.2	– 1.7	2.82
1.4	– 1.6	2.56	1.5	– 1.4	1.96
1.7	– 1.3	1.69	2.1	– 0.8	0.64
3.2	0.2	0.04	2.4	– 0.5	0.25
3.6	0.6	0.36	2.6	0.3	0.09
4.6	1.6	2.56	3.1	0.2	0.04
5.4	2.4	5.76	3.4	0.5	0.25
			4.2	1.3	1.69
			5.2	2.7	7.29
21.0		16.58	26.1		17.10

$$\bar{x}_1 = \frac{\Sigma x_1}{n_1} = \frac{21.0}{7} = 3.0$$

$$\bar{x}_2 = \frac{\Sigma x_2}{n_2} = \frac{26.1}{9} = 2.9$$

$$\sigma_1^2 = \frac{\Sigma(x_1 - \bar{x}_1)^2}{n_2 - 1} = \frac{16.58}{7 - 1} = \frac{16.58}{6} = 2.76$$

$$\sigma_2^2 = \frac{\Sigma(x_2 - \bar{x}_2)^2}{n_2 - 1} = \frac{17.10}{9 - 1} = \frac{17.10}{8} = 2.14$$

$$\therefore \quad = \frac{2.76}{2.14} = 1.29$$

At 5% level of significance, the table value of F for 6 and 8 degrees of freedom is 3.52.

Since 1.29 < 3.52 we conclude that the recovery percentage has not been affected by adjustments in the control panels of the distribution column.

Illustration

Two of random samples were drawn from two normal populations and their values are

A: 65 70 75 76 82 84 88 88 90

B: 90 65 73 72 80 80 88 90 91 93 95

Test whether the two populations have the same variance at the 5% level of significance. (F = 3.11 at 5% level for r_1 = 8 and r_2 = 10)

Solution:

Let us take the hypothesis that the two population, have the same variance.

A.

x_1	$(x_1 - \bar{x}_1) = x_1 - 79.78$	$(x_1 - \bar{x}_1)^2$
65	– 14.78	218.44
70	– 9.78	95.64
75	– 4.78	22.84
76	– 3.78	14.28
82	2.22	4.92
84	4.22	17.80
88	8.22	67.56
88	8.22	67.56
90	10.22	104.44
Total 718	– 0.02	613.48

$$S_1^2 = \frac{\Sigma(x_1 - x_1)^2}{n_1 - 1} = \frac{613.48}{8} = 76.68$$

B.

x_2	$(x_2 - \bar{x}_2) = (x_2 - 80.68)$	$(\bar{x}_2 - \bar{x}_2)^2$ $(x_2 - 80.68)^2$
60	– 20.63	425.59
65	– 15.63	244.29
73	– 7.63	58.21
72	– 8.63	74.47
80	– 0.63	0.39
80	– 0.63	0.39
88	7.37	54.31
90	9.37	87.79
91	10.37	107.53
93	12.37	153.01
95	14.37	206.42
Total 887		1412.54

$$S_2^2 = \frac{\Sigma(x_2 - x_2)^2}{n_2 - 1} = \frac{1412.54}{10} = 141.254$$

$$F = \frac{S_2^2}{S_1^2} = \frac{141.254}{76.68} = 1.842$$

For d.f. $r_1 = 8$ and $r_2 = 10$; F 0.05 = 3.11

YALES CORRELATIONS

One of the conditions for the application of χ^2 test is that no call frequency should be less than 5 in any case, though 10 is better. This requirement is to avoid inflated chi-square values due to the division of the squared differences by a small size of the expected frequency. When the theoretical frequencies are less than 10 and especially less than 5 the ordinary table values of χ^2 are less reliable. This is especially true for one degrees of freedom. It is true to a lesser extent for two or three degree of freedom. However, the error is negligible for more than degree of freedom.

The Yates correction is introduced because the theoretical chi-square distribution is continuous where the tabulated values are based on the distribution of discrete χ^2 statistic. The correction has the effect of reducing the calculated value of χ^2 as compared to the corresponding value without correction.

Types of Errors in Testing Hypothesis

When a statistical hypothesis is tested there are four possibilities

1. The hypothesis is true but our test reject it (Type I error)
2. The hypothesis is false but our test accepts it (Type II error)
3. The hypothesis is true and our test accepts it (Correct decision)
4. The hypothesis is false and our test rejects it (Correct decision).

The first two possibilities lead to errors.

In the context of testing of Hypothesis, there are two types of errors. They are:

Table 5.5: Type I and Type II errors

	Decision	
	Accept H°	Reject H°
H° (True)	Correct decision	Type I α error
H° (False)	Type II β error	Correct decision

In a statistical hypothesis testing experiment, a Type I error is committed by rejecting the null hypothesis when it is true. The probability of committing a Type I error is denoted by a (pronounced as alpha) where

α = Prob. (Type I error)

= Prob. (Rejecting H_0/H_0 is true)

In the other hand a Type II error is committed by not rejecting (i.e., accepting) the null hypothesis when it is false. The probability of committing a Type II error is denoted by β (Pronounced as beta) where

β = Prob. (Type II error)

= Prob. (Not rejecting H_0/H_0 is false)

The distinction between these two types of errors can be made clear by an example. Assume that the difference of two population and sample means is actually zero. If our test of significance, when applied to the two population and sample means, leads us to believe that the difference in population and sample means is significant, we make a Type I error, on the other hand, suppose, there is true difference between the two means, now if our test of significance leads to the judgment "not significant", we commit a Type II error.

While testing hypothesis the aim is to reduce both the types of errors i.e., Type I and Type II. But due to fixed sample size, it is not possible to control both the errors simultaneously. There is a trade off between these types of errors. The probability of making one type of error can only be reduced if we are willing to increase the probability of making the other Type II error. In order to get a low β we will have to put up into a high α.

It is more dangerous to accept false hypothesis (Type II error) than to reject a correct one (Type I error). Hence, we keep the probability of committing Type I error at a certain level, called the level of significance. The level of significance is traditionally denoted by the Greek letter α (pronounced as alpha). In most statistical tests the level of significance is generally fixed at 5%. This means that the probability of accepting a true hypothesis 95%.

Difficulties in The Formulation of Hypothesis

(i) Lack of acquaintance with available research technique resulting in failure to be able to phrase the hypothesis properly.

(ii) Vagueness of the statement, for example, a course in ethics will make a student a more ethical adult.

(iii) Lack of ability to make use of the theoretical framework logically.

(iv) Lack of knowledge and clarity of the theoretical framework of the area in which the investigator chooses to work.

Reference

Dhingra, H.L., *Diversification in Indian Manufacturing Industries.* Punjab University, Supervisor: T.N. Kapur.

CHAPTER 6

Method of Investigation

CENSUS METHOD OF INVESTIGATION

It is very rarely used, specially in case of social phenomena. The most important and large scale census type survey is probably the census of population that is undertaken after regular intervals in every country. In India too census of population is conducted every tenth year. This is the biggest comprehensive study undertaken by the government. In the census of 1951, for example, nearly 7 lakh persons consisting of 6 lakh enumerators and one lakh other supervisory staff, personally visited 644 lakh houses and collected information about 36 crore citizens of the country. Nearly 15 crore rupees were spent on this gigantic venture. These figures were much more higher in 2001.

ADVANTAGES OF CENSUS METHOD

This method is free from sampling errors. There is no chance for personal bias. Highest accuracy is obtained under census method. All the characteristics of the universe is maintained in original.

DISADVANTAGES OF CENSUS METHOD

It involves a great deal of time, money and energy. This method is useless in case results are urgently required. There is possibility for creeping in of statistical errors. A complete enumeration or estimation of all the items in the 'population' may not be necessary.

UNSUITABILITY OF CENSUS METHOD

The very colossal nature method makes it prohibitive to undertake such study. The time, money, and men required for the purpose is very, large, that is it does not seem a practical proposition to undertake such a study, unless it is absolutely essential. Census method, besides the difficulties of time, men and money may create other problems also. It may not be possible at times to know the names of all those concerned, for example, readers of a particular newspaper or users of a particular article. All the person even if known may not be available for contact. They may refuse to meet or their addresses may not be known. Exhaustive and intensive study is also rendered impossible because of the large number. Above all, the sampling enquiry gives significantly correct results with much less time, money, and material. Because of these factors sampling method has received much popularity in surveys and investigations.

SAMPLING METHOD

When a small group is taken as the representative of the whole, the study is called sampling study. The whole group from which the sample has been drawn is technically known as universe or population and the group actually selected for study is known as sample. Sampling is simply the process of learning about population on the basis of a sample drawn from it. Thus, universe and population have to be taken in connection with sampling in entirely different context. According to Prof. Calvin F. Schmid – "a statistical population or universe may consist of attributes, qualities or behaviour of people, the behaviour of inanimate objects such as dice or cities or city blocks, households or dwelling structures, the days output of a factory or opinions or the electorate of an entire nation". "A statistical sample is a miniature picture or cross-section of the entire group or aggregate from which the sample is taken" (P.V. Young).

Objectives of Sampling

The primary objective of the sample survey is to obtain accurate and reliable information about the universe with minimum of cost, time and energy and to set out the limits of accuracy of such estimates.

Basis of Sampling

The choice of a sample as representative of the whole group is based upon certain assumptions :

1. Underlying homogeneity amidst complexity: Although things especially social phenomena, appear to be very complex in nature, so that no two things appear alike, a keener study has disclosed that beneath this apparent diversity, there is underlying fundamental unity. Apparentally ever student may appear to be different. There is difference of health, body, habits, personality etc. but fundamentally they are similar in many respects, so that a study of some of them will throw significant light upon the whole group. It is the possibility of such representative types in the whole population that makes sampling possible. *If no student were alike in any respects the sampling would have been impossible.*

2. Possibility of representative selection: The second assumption is that it is possible to draw a representative sample. It has been proved that if a certain number of units are selected from amass on purely random basis, every unit will have chance of being included and the sample so selected will contain all types of units, so that it may be representative of the whole group. This principle is popularly known as Law of Statistical Regularity and is the very basis of all sampling enquiries.

3. Absolute accuracy not essential: The third basic factor is the fact that absolute accuracy is not essential in case of mass study. In large scale studies we have to depend upon averages which are considered fairly significant in any type of enquiry. Thus, for example, if the average income of a group of a person is Rs. 257 per month. But the sample study discloses it to be 256 or 253. The generalization would not be significantly affected. What material differences does it make whether the income is 256 or 257. Thus, it is not the absolute accuracy but relative or significant accuracy that is needed in case of large scale observation, and the results of sampling studies although not hundred percent accurate are nevertheless sufficiently accurate to permit valid generalizations.

Importance of Sampling in Social Research

Sampling studies are becoming more and more popular in all types of mass studies, but they are specially important in case of social surveys. The vastness of the population, the difficulties of contacting people, high refusal rate, difficulties of ascertaining the universe make sampling the best alternative in case of social studies. The census method is rarely, if ever tried in matters of social research. Recent developments in sampling technique have made this method more reliable and valid. The results of sampling have attained a sufficiently high standard of accuracy. In social research, a close study of the people has to be made, generally taking to sufficiently long period in studying each unit. Under such circumstances sampling is most suitable to be resorted to.

Advantages of Sampling

Sampling method has certain definite advantage over census method. Chief of these advantages are as follows.

1. Saving of time: Comparatively smaller number of units are studied in sampling method and naturally it requires much less time than census method. In certain types of social surveys, time is the most important factor and the result of the study has to be declared quite early to be of any use at all. In all such survey sampling is the only method which can be used.

2. Saving of money: Survey of smaller number of cases not only requires less time, but also requires less money and the study can be financed with much less resources.

3. Detailed study: When the number of units is large, detailed study is not possible. The smaller number of cases in the sample permits a more minute observation and detailed study. In social research, sometimes, a thorough and prolonged study has to be undertaken. This is only possible when the number of cases to be studied is small.

4. Accuracy of result: All the above advantages of sampling are not at the cost of accuracy. On the other hand at times the result drawn by sampling techniques are more reliable than the results from census method. If the sample has been properly selected the results are within a very close range of accuracy. 'Fortune' Magazine of America once made a sample study of 4500 persons to assess the chances in the presidential election. The votes predicted for both the candidates were within 1% error. This shows that if proper *sample is selected the standard of accuracy achieved is sufficiently high.* Techniques have been successfully evolved to calculate the sampling error by means of statistical methods.

5. Administrative convenience: A small sample is usually more convenient from administrative point of view. In social search we have to deal with human beings who cannot be made to work according to our own will. A small sample is, therefore, more manageable specially in social research.

6. Impossibility of the use of census method: In social research the use of census method, sometimes, becomes impossible. It is because the universe is too vast and geographical area is scattered. So that every unit cannot be contacted. Sometimes, the universe is not properly defined as in the case of opinion surveys for a particular product. in such a case it is impossible to know all users of the product and the only method that can be used is the sample method.

Disadvantages of Sampling Method

Following are the main disadvantages of sampling method:

1. Chances of bias: The most common argument against the sampling method is the fact that it may lead to biased selection and thereby leads us to draw false generalizations. A bias in the sample may be caused either by faulty method of sampling or the nature of the phenomena itself.

2. Difficulties of a representative sample: The results of sampling are accurate and usable only when the sample is representative of the whole group. Selection of a completely representative sample is very difficult particularly when the phenomena under the study are of a complex nature as in case of social research.

3. Need for specialized knowledge: The use of sampling method cannot be made by everybody and any body. It requires a specialized knowledge in sampling technique, Statistical analysis, and calculation of probable error. In the absence of such knowledge the researcher may commit untold blunders and entire findings may be reduced to useless scrap.

4. Difficulties in sticking to sample: Although the number of units in the sample is small it is not always easy to stick to it specially in case of social research. The cases of samples may be widely dispersed. Some of them may refuse to co-operate with the researcher, other may be inaccessible, e.g., peregrination ladies. Because of these difficulties complete cases can never be taken up. Sometimes, they have to be replaced by other cases. All these cause a bias in these studies.

5. Impossibilities of sampling: Sometimes, the universe is too small or too heterogeneous so that is impossible to draw a representative sample. In such case census study is the only alternative. In those cases too, where a very high standard of accuracy has to be maintained the sampling method is unsuitable, because even in the most accurate method of sampling, there are always some chances of error.

METHODS OF SAMPLING

(i) Fixed Vs. sequential sampling: Fixed sample involves a predetermined sample size, e.g., a study on "Girl Child and the family", In sequential sampling, the number of units to be sampled is not decided in advance but determined by a decision rule.

(ii) Attributes Vs. variables sampling: (An attribute is a qualitative or descriptive characteristic that a sample unit does or does not possess, e.g., sex. Variables may be any factor including quantitative expression. sampling attempts to estimate a population mean rather than a proportion. (For example, a study on frequency of product purchase).

(iii) Probability Vs. non-probability sampling

TYPES OF SAMPLING

Probability sampling: It provides a scientific techniques of drawing samples from population according to some laws of chance in which each unit has some definite pre-assigned probability of being chosen in the sample. Ramdom sampling, systematic sampling, stratified sampling, cluster sampling, multi-stage sampling and area sampling are considered as probability sampling.

Non-probability sampling or judgment sampling: is based on the personal judgment. Here, a desired number of sample units are selected deliberately or purposely depending upon the object of the enquiry so that only the important items representing the true characteristics of the population are included in the sample. Purposive sampling quota sample and convenience sampling are considered as non-probability sampling.

A number of methods are used for drawing samples, but they can be grouped into the following heads:

1. Random Sampling
2. Purposive Selection
3. Stratified Sampling
4. Quota Sampling
5. Multi-stage Sampling
6. Convenience Sampling
7. Self-selected Sample
8. Systematic sampling.

RANDOM SAMPLING

Of the methods that yield probability samples, simple random sampling is the simplest and one that is basic to all others. Simple random sampling method ensures each of the N units in the population has equal chance or the same chance of being selected. According to Pattern – "Random sampling is the form applied when the method of selection assures each individual or element in universe an equal chance of being chosen". In the words of W.M. Harper, 'A random sample is a sample selected in such a way that every item in the population has an equal chance of being included.' Random sampling is not the same as chance selection. Some people think, if a sample is selected haphazardly without any choice of selection it is always random. It is however, not always so, although in most cases chances selection may prove to be a random selection too. To take an example suppose a page from some book is to be selected at random and for this purpose the book is opened al of a sudden. Now if the book is old, the pages that have been more frequently read will have a greater chance of opening.

Random sampling has also been called proportionate sampling because each class of item is in the same proportion if the sample is in the universe. A random sample is more suitable, more homogenous and comparatively in large groups. When the universe is composed of different groups of extremely varied sizes this method cannot be successfully used. Usually two methods are used to secure true randomness: (i) lottery method is self-explanatory; and (ii) use of random number tables which are published by several authors of whom mention may be made to L.H.G. Tippet (1927), Fisher and Yates (1938), Kendall and Babington Smith (1939).

Methods of Drawing a Random Sample

Following four methods are generally used for drawing out a sample on random basis.

1. Lottery method: Under this system, numbers or names of various units of universe are written on small identical slips of paper which are folded and mixed together in a container thoroughly. A blindfold selection is made. The required number of chits are drawn from the container.

2. Tippet's number: The most practical and economical method of selecting a random sample consists in the use of random numbers which have been so constructed that each of the digits 0, 1,... , 9 appears with approximately the same frequency and independently of each other. One such table of random numbers is constructed by Tippet. L.H.G. Tippet constructed a list of 10400 four digit numbers written at random at every page. They have been constructed out a 41600 digits taken from census reports by combing them in fours. All list of first forty numbers is given below.

Table 6.1: Tippet's Number

2952	6641	3992	9792	7979	5911	3170	5624
4167	9524	545	1396	7203	5356	1300	2693
2370	7483	3408	2762	3563	1089	6913	7691
0560	5246	1112	6107	6008	8126	4433	8776
2754	9143	1405	9025	7002	6111	8816	6446

The method of drawing out the sample from the Tippet's number is very easy. Suppose a sample of 20 person is to be drawn from a list of 6000 persons. For this purpose, first of all we shall number each in it from 0 to 6000. Then we shall open any page of Tippet's numbers and select first twenty numbers that are below 6000. Tippet's numbers are widely used in all the sampling techniques and have been found to be quite reliable as regards accuracy and representativeness.

Selecting from sequential list: Under this plan the names are first arranged according to some particular order which may be alphabetical, geographical or simply serial. Then out of the list every 10th or any other number of case may taken up. A beginning may be made from the middle. Thus, for example, if every tenth from 7th, 17th, 27th, 37th etc. may be selected.

Grid system: It is used for selecting a sample of area. According to this method a map of entire area is prepared. Then a screen with squares are placed upon the map and the areas falling within the selected squares are taken as samples.

Precautions in Drawing a Random Sample

The following precautions should be taken in drawing a random sample:

(i) The population to be sampled should be clearly defined and a list of all units for the purpose of selection should be ready. Different units should be approximately of equal size. Units should be independent of each other and the selection of anyone may not make it binding to select any other unit, e.g., selection of fathers and their sons.

(ii) Every unit should be accessible units. Once selected should not be left out or replaced by other units.

Advantages of Random Sampling

Following are the main advantages of random sampling:

1. It is free from bias and, therefore, not affected by the choice of the researcher.
2. It is generally more representative because *each unit has equal chance of being selected.*
3. It is very simple. The researcher need not exercise his brain in deciding whether a particular unit can be representative or not.
4. Assessment of sampling error can be made. If the sample has been drawn according to strict random sampling basis, it is possible to calculate the limit of error due to sampling.

Disadvantages of Random Sampling

Following are the main advantages of random sampling :

1. It is very difficult to have completely catalogued universe and thus selection according to strictly random basis is frequently not possible. In its place what we generally use is the chance selection.

Cases selected may be too widely dispersed or even impossible to contact and thus adherence to the whole sample may not be possible.

If units are not of different size and the universe consists of many heterogeneous groups of different size, random sampling method is unsuitable.

PURPOSIVE SELECTION/SAMPLING/DELIBERATE SAMPLING/JUDGMENT SAMPLING

When the researcher deliberately or purposively selects certain units for study from the universe, it is known as purposive selection. In this type of sample selection, the choice of the selection is supreme and nothing is left to chance. According to Adolph Jenson – "a purposive selection denotes the method of selecting a number of groups of units in such a way the selected groups together yield as nearly as possible the same averages or proportion as the totality with respect of those characteristics which are already a matter of statistical knowledge".

According to the above definition the following are essential features of purposive selection:

1. The aim of purposive selection is to gain as representative a sample as possible. A representative sample is one which possesses entire qualities of the universe in the same proportion. Following are the criteria of representativeness.
   (a) Different variables are in the same proportion both in the sample as well as in the universe, e.g., proportion of males and females educated, uneducated etc.
   (b) The frequency distribution of the two may be similar.
   (c) Combined average of sample unit is the same as average of universe.
   (d) Variability of the two : sample and universe – is the same. Excepting the first one all other criteria require statistical analysis.
2. In order to achieve the representativeness the selector must possess a complete idea of the nature of universe and various statistical measurements about it.
3. The selector should try to keep himself completely free from any bias. It is better if the samples are selected by more than one person and the common units are taken in selection.

Criticism – According to Parten : "Statisticians as class have nothing to say in favour of purposive selection". Neyman has called this method as hopeless. According to Snedecor there are three main disadvantages of this system:

(a) The knowledge of the population must be available in absence, which is mostly not possible.

(b) The controls are often not effective and a biased sample is selected.

(c) Estimate of sampling error rests upon hypothesis which are seldom met in practice.

In spite of the above criticisms there are some good qualities also. If proper care has been taken in selecting the sample and in keeping out any bias a small sample can be representative of the whole. Thus, purposive selection is at times very cheap. It is more useful specially when some of the units are very important and must be included. Thus, if certain shares are to be selected for constructing sensitive index numbers, random sampling can be resorted to as some of the shares must be included in the list if it is to be at all representative.

STRATIFIED SAMPLING

Stratification means division of the universe into groups according to geographical, sociological or economic characteristics. It is a combination of both random sampling and purposive selection. Under this system the universe is first divided into a number of strata or groups. Then from each group certain number of items are taken on random basis. Thus, in the selection of strata we use purposive selection method, but in selecting actual units from each stratum random method is used.

Process of Stratifying

The source of stratified sampling depends upon formation of strata or groups. If a correct stratification has been made even a smaller number of units will form a representative sample. Following points may be kept in mind while constructing strata:

1. First of all we should note the different variables involved and used in the study of the problem. The common variables used for stratification are generally region, income, sex etc. The universe is first divided into groups and then the required units are selected at random from each group. In selecting the variables, care should be taken to see that they are related to study.
2. The size of each stratum in the universe should be large enough to provide selection of items on random basis. If the strata are too small, difficulty may be created in making a random selection.
3. Stratification should be so conducted that there should be perfect homogeneity in the different units of strata. The items in one stratum should be similar to each other but they should differ significantly from the units of other strata.

4. It is desirable that number of items to be selected from each stratum should be in the same ratio to the total number of units in the stratum the same ratio. In a certain social group it is 75%, the same percentage of units will be selected from amongst the educated.
5. The strata should be clear cut and free from overlapping, so that every unit must find a place in some stratum or the other and no unit should be placed in more than one stratum. The total number of units in different strata should be equal to total number of units in universe.

Kinds of Stratified Sampling

Stratified sampling itself is of the following three types:

(1) **Proportional stratified sample:** In method the number of units to be drawn from each stratum is in the same proportion as they stand in the universe. It has already been explained above.

(2) **Disproportional stratified sample:** According to this method an equal number of cases are taken from each stratum regardless of the size of strata in proportion in the universe. It is also known as controlled sampling because it permits inter-strata comparison.

(3) **Stratified weighted sampling:** This method aims as removing the defects of disproportion sample and combine the advantages of the two stratified samples stated earlier. The disproportion sample has one defect, that it creates bias over weighting some of the strata. In this system equal number of units are selected from each stratum. Averages are taken from each stratum but they are given weights in proportion to the size of stratum in the whole universe.

Advantages of Stratified Sampling

Following are the main advantages of stratified sampling:

1. The sampler gets a greater control over the sample. In random sample although every unit has an equal chance of being selected, sometimes, important groups are left out by chance. Under stratified sampling no significant group is left unrepresented.
2. If proper stratification has been made a representative character can be achieved with fewer items. If a stratum is perfectly homogeneous, selection of even a few items from it is enough.
3. Replacement of case can be resorted too easily if the original case is no accessible to study. If a person refuses to co-operate with the survey, h may be replaced by another man from the same stratum.
4. In stratification, the sample can be so selected that most of the units ar geographically localized. In a purely random sample there is not enoug

control and the cases actually selected may be very widely dispersed. Concentration of units saves time and cost of survey.

5. It is of great help if the distribution of the universe is skewed.
6. It is the only sampling plan which enables us to achieve different degrees of accuracy for different segments of the population.
7. Stratified random sampling is more precise and to a great extent avoids bias. It also saves time and cost of data collection since the sample size can be less in this method.

Disadvantages of Stratified Sampling

Following are the main disadvantages of stratified sampling:

1. Bias may be caused in the sample through improper stratification. If the strata are overlapping, unsuitable for the problem under study or disproportionate, the selection of the sample may not be representative.
2. A sample in order to be representative must be proportionate. Proportion is attained in random sampling. Automatically in stratified sampling deliberate attempt has to be made in this respect. Attainment of proportion is very difficult through deliberate means specially when of the size of different strata is extremely unequal.
3. Disproportionate stratification requires weighting which again introduces selective factor in the sample. An undue weighting makes the sample unrepresentative.
4. Difficulty may be experienced in putting particular case in a stratum. If the strata are not very clear cut it may be difficult to decide in which stratum any particular unit is to be placed.

QUOTA SAMPLING

Quota sampling is a special type of stratified sampling. According to this method the universe is first divided into different strata. Then the number to be selected from each stratum is decided. This number is known as the quota. The field workers are generally asked to select the quota from the stratum according to their will. To take an example supposes a sample of 500 families is to be selected. Under this system, the houses to be approached will be decided first and the field workers will be asked to select one family from each house at their will. Quota sampling is a stratified-cum-purposive sampling and thus enjoys the benefits of both above named methods. It makes the best use of stratification economically. It is only useful method when no sample frame is available. However, this method suffers from the limitations of both stratified and purposive sampling. Bias may also occur due to substitution of unlike sample units. Moreover, sampling error and standard error cannot be estimated.

Multi-stage Sampling

This method is generally used in selecting a sample from very large area. Under this method the selection of the sample is made in various stages. For example, the following procedure would be adopted to select a sample of a few hundred houses from a large city.

(a) Divide the whole city into homogeneous regions. Care should be taken to see that each region is approximately equal in size and there is similarity among the people of one region at least regarding the aspect that is being studied.

(b) Select two primary sample areas from each region or random sampling method.

(c) Select one block cluster (group of houses) from primary sample area.

(d) Select some houses from each block cluster on random sampling basis.

Thus, we see that the selection of final sample units is made in a number of stages. The method is thus a combination of random sampling and stratified sampling, and if conducted judiciously it possess the advantages of both the types. Greater representation can be achieved in shortest possible numbers and representation of every area is secured. Multi-stage sampling is more flexible in comparison to the other methods of sampling. This technique is of great significance in surveys of underdeveloped areas where no up to date and accurate frame is generally available for sub-division of the materials into reasonably small sampling units. Under this method surveys can be conducted with considerable speed. However, errors are likely to be large in this method in comparison to any other method. It involves considerable amount of listing of first stage units, second stage units etc., though complete listing of units is not necessary.

Convenience Sampling

It is generally known as unsystematic, careless, accidental or opportunistic sampling. According to this system, a sample is selected according to the convenience of the sampler. This convenience may be in respect of availability of source list, accessibility of the units etc. Although the method is most unscientific, yet quite a large number of samples are selected according to this method. A convenience sampling may be used in any one or more of the following cases:

(a) When the universe is not clearly defined.

(b) When sampling unit is not clear.

(c) When a complete source list is not available.

Thus, the selection of names from telephone directory, Industrial or Stock Exchange Directories, Automobile Registration Records will come under this type of sampling.

Self-selected Sample

Sometimes, a sample is not actually selected but people themselves opt to be included or not to be included in a sample. Suppose, for example, an enquiry has to be made about the people's liking for a particular radio programme, and an announcement to this effect is made on the radio, in such case, the sample is not fixed. Those who care to reply form the part of the sample. Such a sample is known as self-selected sample.

Cluster Sampling

Under this method, the total population is divided into some recognizable sub-divisions which are termed as clusters and a simple random sample of these clusters is drawn and then the survey of each and every unit in the selected cluster is made.

Principles of Cluster Sampling

- Cluster should be as small as possible with the cost and limitations of the survey.
- The number of sampling units in each cluster should be approximately same.

Merits: This method provides significant cost gain and it is easier and more practical method which facilitates the field work.

Demerits: The results obtained under this method are likely to be less accurate if the numbers of sampling units in each cluster are not approximately the same.

Systematic Sampling

Under this method a sample is taken from a list prepared on the basis of alphabetic order or on house number or any other method. In this method, only the first sample unit is selected at random and the remaining units are automatically selected in a definite sequence at equal spacing from one another.

Types of Purposeful Sampling

(i) Convenience sampling
(ii) Critical case sampling
(iii) Extreme case sampling
(iv) Homogeneous sampling
(v) Intensity sampling
(vi) Maximum variation sampling
(vii) Purposeful random sampling
(viii) Snowball or network sampling
(ix) Typical case sampling
(x) Theory-based sampling.

Other Sampling Methods

Snow Ball Sampling

This method is used where the information about units within the population is not available. For instance, if the researcher wants to study the problems faced by Indians in the City of New York, he would contact all the Indians in the City of New York who could be located. Those contacted would be asked to give the names of other Indians in the City of New York. By repeating the process in several stages a majority of Indians in the City of New York could hopefully be identified and contacted. From this group a sample would be drawn.

Spatial Sampling

Some population move from place to place. In such a case, the whole population (wherever possible) at a particular place are taken into the sampling and studied.

Saturation Sampling

It requires a study of all population. In sociometric studies, this technique is adopted. In such studies even if one person is left out, we get distorted results.

HOW TO SELECT A SAMPLE

The procedure of selecting a sample differs according to the type of sample selected. Yet certain fundamental rules can be cited. Following steps are generally taken in selecting the sample:

(1) Defining Universe: The whole group from which the sample is to be selected is technically called universe or population. Thus, in order to draw the sample we must first of all have a clear idea of the universe from which the sample is to be drawn. In some cases, the universe has the geographical limits and then it is very easy to locate it. But if the universe depends upon some quality or attribute, definition of the universe becomes rather difficult.

Thus, for example, if an opinion survey about a particular radio programme is to be made the universe will consist of all those people who have listened to that programme. Naturally it is would be difficult task to define such an universe.

Different types of Universe : The universe from which the sample is to be drawn may be classified into following types:

(a) **Definite and indefinite universe:** When the number of units falling within the universe can be definitely ascertained it is known as definite universe, e.g., a city or locality or students of a college or university. When this number and the exact units cannot be ascertained we call it indefinite universe. An universe may be indefinite because of its constantly changing nature like young babies. Their number cannot be ascertained over a period of time as these numbers are constantly changing. If may be indefinite when the cases cannot be located, e.g., the users of a particular radio programme.

(b) **Real and hypothetical universe:** The universe may be a real or simply hypothetical. Hypothetical universe is not used in case of surveys. But it has great utility in statistical analysis. Most of the statistical generalizations are made from a purely hypothetical universe. Thus, for example, after studying the census of population we may draw certain mathematical formulae regarding the distribution of population in different age groups. Now if the total population of a place falling within a similar class is given to us we can form a theoretical frequency distribution of various age groups and thus determine the number of units to be drawn from each group. This type of universe will be known as hypothetical universe.

(2) **Sampling Unit:** Before drawing a sampling we have to decide the unit of sample. What shall we select: a house, a family, an individual or a group surveyors have fallen into the error of thinking that as long as they are dealing with human population, the individual persons are the sampling units actually; however, relatively few studies have used people as sampling units.

Following are the main types of sampling units.

(a) Geographical units – e.g., a state, district, city, ward, region or locality.

(b) Structural units – e.g., a house, a flat etc.

(c) Social group units – e.g., a family a school, a club, a church, etc.

(d) Individuals.

The house or residential dwelling is generally considered as the best unit in the sense that it can be easily located.

Qualities of a good unit : Following are the main qualities of a good sampling unit.

1. The unit should be clear, unambiguous and definite. It should be capable of being objectively ascertained and easily located. Thus, for example, 'an honest man is not a fit unit as it is difficult to be ascertained.

2. The unit of sample should be suitable for the problem under study. Thus in study of the influence of joint family system, family will be the most suitable unit.

3. The unit selected should be standardized if possible if an entirely new unit has been used, its meaning and significance should be explained clearly.

4. The unit should be easily ascertainable. Thus, if an individual is to be selected as unit, it is difficult to find the names of all the individuals concerned and even if they are known, it is very difficult to find them unless their names are accompanied with their addresses.

Source List

The list which contains the name of the units of universe from which the sample is to be selected is technically known as source list. A source list may be already in existence or it may have to be prepared. For example, names of all the house owners, telephone owners etc., can be seen from list maintained by respective departments. But the list of the tenants occupying particular area or house has to be prepared. Sometimes, the list may be available in parts and may have to be consolidated. At other times, the list may be exhaustive and relevant. Universe may have to be sorted out.

Qualities of a usable source list: The following points are worth noting before using the source list:

1. The list should be exhaustive. The entire universe to be studied must be contained in the source list.
2. The list should be up to date and valid. It should not contain dead names and must include the latest additions to the list.
3. The list should contain full information about the units so that the sample may be drawn on stratified basis. It should contain the addresses also so that it may be possible to contact the units selected.
4. The names should not be repeated in the list. For example, if the list of guardians is maintained, the name of a person may be found at more than one places according to the number of school going children.

5. The source list should be suitable for the unit of study. For example, if any family has been selected as unit, the list containing individual names for house numbers would be of no value.
6. Source list must be reliable. It must be maintained by an authority that can be relied upon.
7. Source list must be written by the researcher. Thus, for example, the government may maintain a list of history sheets but it may not be kept open for the public. Similarly, a bank although, maintaining a list of depositors may refuse to supply it to the researcher. Such lists are to be released when a survey is to be conducted by the same department or under the authority of the government.

SIZE OF SAMPLE

The size of the sample is an important problem to be decided in case of sampling. This is because the size has a direct bearing upon accuracy, time, cost, and administration of the survey. Large samples are generally hard to manage and are unfit for detailed study, but that may be essential for representativeness. According to Parten – "An optimum sample in survey is one which fulfills the requirements of efficiency, representativeness, reliability and flexibility". The sample should be small enough to avoid unnecessary expenses and large enough to avoid intolerable sampling error.

FACTORS AFFECTING THE SIZE OF THE SAMPLE

The size of the sample depends upon a number of factors, the chief of which are stated below:

1. **Homogeneity or heterogeneity of universe:** If the universe is comparatively homogeneous a smaller size of the sample may be sufficient. If all the units were exactly alike one single unit could serve as sample, but if the universe is heterogeneous, so that very few units are similar, the sample has to be essentially larger in size.
2. **Number of classes proposed:** If a large number of classes are to be formed the sample must be large enough, so that every class may be of proper size suitable for statistical treatment. If the size of the sample is small there may be some classes which may contain one or two units only. Some may remain totally unrepresented. The result is that they cannot be analyzed properly and the generalization based upon them will also not be correct. Thus, larger the number of classes proposed greater will be the size of the sample.

3. **Nature of study:** The size of the sample will also depend upon the nature of study. If an intensive study is to be made continuously for a pretty long time, large sample is unfit for the purpose as it will require very large finance and other resources. Thus, in case of opinion surveys where people have to be contacted for knowing their opinion about the problem under the study the interview is quite short and much larger number of units may be included in the sample. Similarly, in case of general study large number of cases at can be taken but if the study is of a technical nature a large number may become difficult to manage.
4. **Practical considerations:** Practical considerations as availability of finance, time at our disposal, number of trained field workers etc., may also be taken as important factor in deciding the size of the sample. The limitations of these resources necessarily limit the size of the sample. One thing must be made clear at this stage. Although these practical considerations do weigh heavily in determining the size of the sample it should never be done at the cost of accuracy. Any amount of money, how so ever small, spent on an unrepresentative sample, is pure and simple waste and must be avoided at all cost.
5. **Standard of accuracy:** It is generally considered that larger the size of the sample greater is the standard of accuracy or representativeness. Although this is not true in all cases, as mere largeness of size is no guarantee for representativeness. A small but well selected sample may give better results than a larger and thoughtlessly selected sample. National Opinion Research Centre (N.O.R.C.), the premier opinion survey agency of America, is now turning more and more to small size samples. In 1946 N.O.R.C. selected about 2500 cases in a standard poll. In 1948 it was reduced to 1300 cases only. As the technique of sampling is becoming more and more scientific and refined better standard of accuracy has been possible to be achieved by comparatively smaller samples.

   In spite of the above argument, the general fact remains that larger sample is necessary for greater reliability. A short sample can only be reliable when it has been drawn by experts and in very favourable circumstances. But that is not always possible. No guidance is generally available for drawing sample. There are other limitations like inadequate source list, lack of complete knowledge about the universe, and the units of which it composed one under these limitations. It is always safer to draw comparatively larger sample to make it more reliable and representative.
6. **Size of the questionnaire or schedule:** The size of the questionnaire and the nature of questions to be asked is also a limiting factor for the size of the sample. Larger the size of schedule more complicated the questions to be asked. Smaller is to be the size for proper administration.

7. **Nature of cases to be contacted:** The nature of cases to be contacted plays its own part in deciding the size of the sample. If the cases are geographically scattered a small sample is more suitable. On the other hand, if the refusal rate is likely to be heavy or losses of cases likely to be quite big, a larger sample has to be selected, so that after providing for the cases who may refuse to reply or those that may not be available due to other cause, the actual number of cases that is left out may be large enough to permit statistical analysis.
8. **Type of sampling used:** If absolute random sampling has been used much larger sample is required. Random sample is reliable only when sufficiently large sample units are used. Because it is only in large number of cases that law of statistical regularity properly works and every class of unit gets a chance of being selected. On the other hand, if the stratified sample has been selected, reliability can be achieved in a much smaller size. But in stratified sampling the essential conditions are that stratification must be proper. If stratification is unsuitable and improper a large number will only add to the bias in the sample.

These are some of broad considerations that are to be kept in mind. In fact no rigid number can be prescribed for an optimum size of the sample. The nature of the problem is the only deciding factor and the common sense and experience of the researcher the only guide in this matter.

FORMULAE FOR SAMPLE SIZE

Mildred Parten has given the following formula for calculating sample size.

$$\text{Sample size} = \left(\frac{SZ}{T}\right)$$

where S stands for the preliminary standard deviation of the universe.

Z stands for the number of standard error units.

T stands for the margin of error to be tolerated.

In the formula used for determining sample size, a prior estimate of the standard deviation of the population and level of confidence is necessary. The confidence level is taken 95% or 99%.

MINIMUM SAMPLE SIZE

The following formula can be used to determine the minimum size of the sample:

$$\sqrt{n} = \frac{(1.96)(\sigma)}{\text{Prevision}} \quad \text{or} \quad n = \left[\frac{(1.96)(\sigma)}{\text{Prevision}}\right]^2$$

In this formula, n = sample size, 1.96 = 95% confidence level,

σ = population standard deviation.

TESTING RELIABILITY OF SAMPLE

The researcher must make sure that the sample selected by him is reliable or representative and valid generalization can be drawn from it. The following methods are generally adopted for testing the reliability of the sample:

1. **By drawing a parallel sample:** Another sample may be drawn from the same universe and if various measurements viz., average, dispersion, frequency distribution are taken are identicaly. The readers must know at this point that no two samples, howsoever, accurately drawn, can be exactly alike. They are significantly alike. A mathematical measurement known as sampling error or standard error is adopted for this purpose.
2. **By comparing the measurement of the sample with those of the universe if known:** Sometimes, the different measurements of the universe are known, e.g., equality of sex ratio, age distribution etc. In such cases, the various measurements of the sample are compared with those of the universe and if the difference is significant the sample is considered to be unrepresentative or biased.
3. **By drawing a sub sample from the main sample:** Sometimes, sub-sample from the main sample is selected. It is intensively studied and the findings are compared with the main sample. This method is not used for testing the representativeness of the sample but to detect any error that might have crept in due to faulty collection of facts.

USE OF SAMPLING IN SOCIAL RESEARCH

The use of sampling methods has been very old in social research. According to Stephen they were used even earlier than census method. As early as in 1754, the census of population of England was conducted by this method. According to this method average number of people living in a house was assumed to be 6 and total population was calculated by multiplying the number of houses with 6. In 1800 also the same method was used, but this time average number of births was added to it.

In 1936, B.S., Rowntree made a detailed study of working class conditions in the city of New York. He first of all contacted 19362 families. Later on he tried the sampling method to test its reliability. He first of all selected every tenth houses, thus, taking a sample of 1936 houses. He also took subsequent samples selecting very 20th, 30th, 40th and 50th houses. Thus, he undertook five sample studies of the same population every time reducing the sample. His findings were that the results of sampling were quite reliable. According to census type study 31% of the population was living a life below standard. In case of sample it was between 31.1 to 33.1%.

It was Prof. A.L. Bowley who first of all introduced the principle of random sampling in social research. He conducted his study in collaboration with Burnett Hurst to compare the incidence of poverty at different times and places. They visited one in every 20 houses at random. Bowley gave a very elaborate treatise of random sampling and the methods of calculating the standard errors. Snedecor was so much impressed by Bowley's work that at one place he goes on to say – "Bowley's monumental investigation of mathematical theory of representative sampling has since been improved in minor details, with a few notable exceptions, it may be said that most of our present knowledge of sampling of social facts is explained in the Journal of the International Institute".

Since that time there has been constant improvement in the sampling technique, methods of calculating the probable errors etc., more and more use has been made of the sampling technique in social researches, surveys and polls, In fact, social research has been possible only through sampling method.

ERRORS IN SAMPLING

I. SAMPLING ERRORS

Meaning: According to Patterson, "Sampling error is the difference between the result of studying a sample and inferring a result about the population and the result of the census of the whole population". Sampling errors are the random variables in the sample estimates around the true population parameters. Since they occur randomly and are equally likely to be in either direction, their nature happens to be of compensatory type and the expected value of such error happens to be equal to zero. Sampling error decreases with the increase in the size of the sample (number of units selected in the samples) and it happens to be of a smaller magnitude in case of homogeneous population. In many situations, the sampling error is approximately inversely proportional to the square-root of the number of units included in the sample. It can be represented in the form of a diagram. We measure sampling error in the y-axis and the sample size in the x-axis. And the curve is negative in slope (like a demand curve). See Fig. 6.1 "Reducing sampling error".

Types: Sampling errors are of two types Biased and Unbiased Errors.

Biased Errors

Biased errors are those which arise as a result of any bias or prejudice of the person in selecting a particular sampling method. For example, purposive and deliberate sampling method may be adopted in place of a simple random sampling method. As a result of such a selection, some errors are bound to arise. And they are known as biased errors. Such errors are also known as cumulative errors or non-compensating errors.

These are the errors which arise from any bias in selection estimation etc., for example, if in place of simple random sampling, deliberate sampling has been used in a particular case some bias is introduced in the result and hence, such errors are called biased errors.

Causes of Bias

Bias in sampling may arise under the following circumstances:

1. Faulty process of sample selection
2. Faulty methods of data collection
3. Faulty methods of analysis.

Unbiased Errors

Unbiased errors are such errors which are either accidental or arise in the natural course of events and are without any bias or prejudice. They arise because of chance difference between the members of population included in the sample and those not included. It is also known as random errors. These are the errors which arise due to chance difference between the number of population included in the population and those not included.

II. Non-Sampling Errors

Meaning: According to Patterson: "Non-sampling errors are errors that occur in acquiring, recording, or tabulating statistical data that cannot be described to sampling error. They may arise in either a census or a sample".

Types (Causes) of Non-sampling Errors: Non-sampling errors are caused by the following:

- Faulty problem definitions
- Defective population definition
- Inadequate and inconsistent data specification
- Inappropriate statistical unit
- Inaccurate or inappropriate methods of data collection
- Lack of trained and experienced investigators
- Lack of adequate inspection and supervision of primary staff
- Frame is non-representative of the population
- Non-response errors
- Measurement error
- Poor questionnaire design
- Improper causal inferences
- Interpretation errors

- Data processing errors
- Data analysis errors
- Errors due to non-response caused by incomplete coverage of units
- Error in data processing operations such as coding, punching, verification etc.
- Errors committed during presentation and printing of tabulating results.
- They occur due to the use of sampling surveys. Even when a sample is random one, it may not be exactly representative of the population from which it is chosen. Samples may be taken from the same population four times. All samples may not be alike. This also gives rise to sampling errors.
- Total Error = Sampling Error + Non-sampling Error.

Methods of Reducing Sampling Error

The sampling errors must be reduced to the minimum, so that the results and conclusions are sufficiently representative of the whole universe. This can be done by removing errors of bias from the sample and by enlarging the size of the sample. The sampling error is approximately inversely proportional to the square-root of the number of units included in the sample, as represented in the following figure:

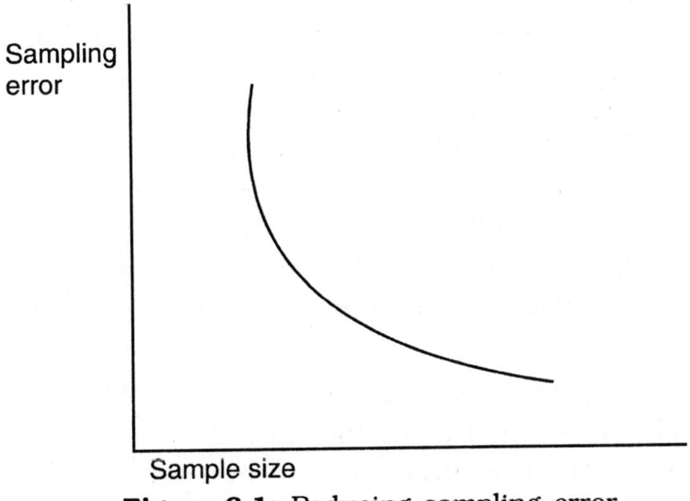

Figure 6.1: Reducing sampling error.

Reducing sampling error is initially possible by increasing the size of the sample but it becomes marginal after a certain stage.

Correlation, Probable and Standard Errors

Sources of Errors

(i) Use of inappropriate average or wrong use of average
(ii) Drawing unwarranted conclusions
(iii) Irrelevant data
(iv) Unequal basis of comparison
(v) Drawing inferences from an argument running from effect to cause
(vi) False generalizations
(vii) Coefficient of association is also often responsible for wrong interpretation
(viii) Percentages are commonly responsible for erroneous conclusions.

Methods of Studying Correlation:

The various methods of ascertaining whether two variables are correlated or not are:

I. Scatter Diagram Method
II. Graphic Method
III. Karl Pearson's Coefficient of Correlation
IV. Concurrent Deviation Method
V. Method of Least Squares.

Of these, the first two are based on the knowledge of diagram and graphs, whereas others are the mathematical methods.

Interpreting Coefficient of Correlation

The coefficient of correlation measures the degree of relationship between two sets of figures. As the reliability of estimates depends upon the closeness of the relationship, it is imperative that utmost care be taken while interpreting the value of coefficient of correlation, otherwise fallacious conclusions can be drawn.

Unfortunately, the interpretation of the coefficient of correlation "r" depends very much on experience. The full significance of "r" will only be grasped after working out a number of correlation problems and seeing the kinds of data that gives rise to various values of "r". The investigator must know his data thoroughly in order to avoid errors of interpretation and emphasis. He must be familiar, or become familiar, with all the relationships and theory which bear upon the data and should reach a conclusion based on logical reasoning and intelligence investigation on significantly related matters. However, the following general rules are given which would help in interpreting the value of "r".

1. When r = +1, it means there is perfect positive relationship between the variables.
2. When r = −1, it means there is perfect negative relationship between the variables.
3. When r = 0, it means that there is no relationship between the variable, i.e., the variables are uncorrelated.
4. The closer r is to +1 or −1, the closer the relationship between the variables and closer r is to 0, the less close the relationship. Beyond this it is not safe to go. The full interpretation of r depends upon circumstances, one of which is the size of the sample. All that can really be said that when estimating the value of one variable from the value of another, the higher the value of r, the better the estimates.
5. The closeness of the relationship is not proportional to r. If the value of r is 0.8, it does not indicate a relationship twice as close as one of 0.4. It is, in fact, very much closer.

COEFFICIENT OF CORRELATION AND PROBABLE ERROR

The probable error of the coefficient of correlation helps in interpreting its value. With the help of probable error it is possible to determine the reliability of the value of the coefficient in so far as it depends on the conditions of random sampling. The probable error of the coefficient of correlation is obtained as follows:

$$\text{P.E.} = 0.6745\ \frac{1 - r^2}{\sqrt{N}}$$

where r is the coefficient of correlation and N the number of pairs of observation.

1. If the value of r is less than the probable error there is no evidence of correlation, i.e., the value of r is not at all significant.
2. If the value of r is more than six times the probable error, the coefficient of correlation is practically certain, i.e., the value of r is significant.
3. By adding and substracting the value of probable error from the coefficient of correlation we get respectively the upper and lower limits within which coefficient of correlation in the population can be expected to lie. Symbolically,

$$P = \rho \pm \text{P.E.}$$

Where ρ (rho) denotes correlation in the population and N = 6

Let us compute probable error, assuming a coefficient of correlation of 0.80 and a sample of pairs of items. We will have

$$\text{P.E.} = 0.6745 \frac{1-(.8)^2}{\sqrt{16}}$$

If 0.6745 is omitted from the formula of probable error, we get the standard error of the coefficient of correlation. The standard error ρ therefore is:

$$\text{S.E.} = \frac{1-\rho^2}{\sqrt{N}}$$

The limits of the correlation in the population would be ρ + P.E., i.e., 0.8 + 0.06 or 0.74 – 0.86.

Instances are quite common wherein a correlation coefficient of 0.5 or even 0.4 is obiviously considered to be fairly high degree of correlation by a writer or research worker. Yet, a correct coefficient of 0.5 means that only 25 per cent of the variation is explained. A correlation coefficient of 0.4 means that only 16 per cent of the variation is explained.

Conditions for the Use of Probable Error:

The measure of probable error can be probably used only when the following three conditions exist:

1. The data must approximately be a normal frequency curve (bell-shaped curve).
2. The statistical measure for which the P.E. is computed must have been calculated from a sample.
3. The sample must have been selected in an unbiased manner and the individual items must be independent.

However, these conditions are generally satisfied and as such the reliability of the correlation coefficient is determined largely on the basis of exterior tests of reasonableness which are often of a statistical character.

STANDARD ERROR OF ESTIMATE

With the help of regression equations perfect prediction is practically impossible. For example, the revenue for the year from gasoline sales (y) based on automobile registered (x) as of a certain date would no doubt be approximately fairly closely, but prediction may not be exact to the nearest rupee nor probably to the nearest 1000 rupees. What is needed, then, is a measure, which would indicate how precise the prediction of y is, based on x or conversely, how accurate the prediction might be. The measure is called the standard error of estimate. The standard error of estimate is symbolized by S_{yx}. The standard deviation measures the dispersion about an average, such as the mean. The standard error of estimate measures the dispersion about an average line, called the regression line. The formula for calculating the standard error of estimate is

$$S_{yx} = \sqrt{\frac{\Sigma(Y - Y)_c^{\,2}}{N}} \quad \text{i.e.,} \quad \sqrt{\frac{\text{Unexplained Variation}}{N}}$$

Also $\quad S_{yx} = \sigma_y\sqrt{1 - r^2}$

where $\quad S_{yx}$ = the standard error of regression of Y values from Y_c.

This formulation is not convenient from the computational point of view because it requires the computation of $(Y - Y_c)$. A more convenient formula is

$$S_{yx} = \sqrt{\frac{\Sigma Y^2 - a\Sigma y - b\Sigma xy}{N}}$$

The standard error of regression of X value from X_c is

$$S_{yx} = \sqrt{\frac{\Sigma(X - X_c)^2}{N}} \quad \text{also } S_{yx} = \sigma_x\sqrt{1 - r^2}$$

Also

$$S_{yx} = \sqrt{\frac{\Sigma X^2 - a\Sigma X - b\Sigma xy}{N}}$$

S_{yx} = the standard of regression of X values from X_c.

The standard error of estimate measures the accuracy of the estimated figures. The smaller the value of standard error of estimate, the closer will be dots to the regression line and the better the estimates based on the equation for this line. If the standard error of estimate is zero, then there is no variation about the line and the correlation will be perfect. Thus, with the help of standard error estimate, it is possible for us to ascertain how good and representative the regression line is as a description of the average relationship between two series.

Compound Interest Formula

$$P_n = P_0\,(1 + r)^n$$

where, $\quad P_0$ = the amount at the beginning of the period

P_n = The amount at the end of the period

r = Rate of change

n = Number of time periods.

It follows from the above formula that

$$r = \sqrt{\frac{P_n}{P_0}} - 1$$

$$P_n = P_0(1 + r)^n$$

STANDARD ERROR

The standard deviations of the sampling distribution is called the standard error. For example, x_1, x_2, ... etc., are the means of all the samples drawn from the population, the standard deviations of all these means is the standard error of the mean.

CHAPTER 7 Observation

MEANING

Observation means acquiring knowledge through the use of sense organs. It implies the use of eyes rather than the ears and the voice. Observation is systematic and deliberate study through the eye of spontaneous occurrences as they occur. The Oxford Concise Dictionary defines Observation as 'accurate watching and nothing of phenomena as they occur in nature with regard to cause and effect or mutual relations'. Dr. P.V. Young defines Observation as 'a systematic and deliberate study through the eye of spontaneous occurrences at the time they occur'. It is a systematic viewing coupled with consideration of the seen phenomena. It is a deliberate study through the eye, which may be used as one of the methods for scrutinizing collective behaviour and complex of institutions as well as separate units composing of totality. According to Goode and Hatt, observation includes the most casual uncontrolled experiences as well as the most exact film records of laboratory experimentation. Observation is defined as the process of recognizing and noting people, objects and occurrences rather than asking for information. Under the Observation method the information is sought by way of investigators' own direct Observation without asking from the respondent. Observation seeks to ascertain the external behaviour of persons in a variety of situations. The external behaviour of persons in a variety of situations are both controlled or uncontrolled.

Observation a scientific technique: Science begins with Observation and must ultimately return to Observation for its final validation. Observation becomes a scientific technique to the extent that it:

- It serves a formulated research purpose.
- It is planned systematically.
- It is corded systematically and related to more general propositions.
- It is subjected to checks and controls on validity and reliability.

Components of Observation

There are three important components of observations:

1. Sensation,
2. Attention, and
3. Perception.

General Characteristics of Observation Method

Observation, as a technique of data collection, has the following general characteristics:

Physical and mental activity: Observation involves the use of sense organs of the investigator. He has to see or hear the thing and then keep it in mind or record the same for careful analysis at a later stage.

Specific, selective and purposeful: A researcher selects his area of activity and the things he is required to observe. Then only, it becomes a purposeful research affair. Observation is guided by distinct motives or gainful purposes.

Tools of research: If it is to be finally useful, Observation should be based on scientific tools of research which have been fairly standardized.

Direct study: This is a scientific method where the researcher makes a direct study of the situation or phenomenon. It is, in fact, the only method for collecting reliable primary data.

Cause and effect relationships: This method tries to establish a logical relationship between the cause and effect in the observed phenomenon.

Systematic and scientific: Intelligent planning, expert execution, adequate recording, and, scientific interpretation are various steps involved in a scientific and systematic Observation.

Observation is expert: Observation is expert, that is, done by a specially well-trained person for a distinct purposes.

Observation is quantitative: Observation is usually with a tally of the number of instances that a particular type of behaviour has occurred.

Carefully noted: All occurrences have to be carefully noted either at the time of Observation or immediately after the Observation. The social investigator uses recording devices such as check lists, rating scales, score cards, sealed specimen, and blank forms for tallying frequencies. The use of well constructed proforma helps in summarizing and quantifying of the data collected by Observation.

Subjects to checks and verification: The results of all systematic observation are subjected to checks and verification.

Relation with Hypothesis (H)

Observation is a logical start in the formulation of hypothesis. The researcher first observes a thing and then forms his opinion which is developed later as a hypothesis. For instance one may tentatively formulate an exploratory hypothesis that accidents are caused by speeding vehicles. In this context, case study may be designed to focus on the speeding vehicles and the consequences of such speed.

Observation as a Technique of Data Collection

As Goode and Hatt rightly put science begins with Observation. Copernicus has observed the things which have occurred during his time. Even today, Observation is the touch stone of scientific activity in establishing the cause and effect relationship. Observation proved to be an important technique of conducting research in physical, natural and social sciences. Observation is, perhaps, the only method perfectly suited to study the behaviour of social phenomena. Observation is the only way through which the child accumulates knowledge uses it for future retrieval.

As regards social sciences. Observation is the most commonly used method in collecting data regarding the behaviour of human beings of a social phenomena. In the studies like consumer behaviour, executive behaviour, and workers behaviour, Observation proves to be a very good technique of data collection. In the fields of commerce and economics, observation of the prices, markets, and capital flows is more a common activity which serves as a good, e.g., for probing into the behaviour of the phenomena. Observation is considered to be a handy tool in marketing research. Some of the major studies in consumer behaviour in the U.S.A. are conducted with the help of Observation. In some cases, Observation is considered to be the only way to obtain marketing information required for the study. For example, if a store manager wishes to determine the current pricing and sales promotion activity taking place at his competitors establishment, a personal visit may be necessary. Such casual Observation, while providing useful information, would enable him to get first-hand account of the situation.

PROCESS OF OBSERVATION

Observation is a sequential process which helps the researcher to record results with precision. Lin Naw in his 'Foundation of social Research' has identified five sequential steps in the observation method. They are: (i) Preparation and training, (ii) Entry into the study environment, (iii) Initial interaction, (iv) Observations and recording, and (v) Termination of field work.

1. **Preparation and training:** The researcher must decide what, where and how to observe the thing. He should prepare the necessary ground for Observation. For example, the researcher is interested in observing the morals and commitment of the workers in a factory. In this context, he has to decide whether he is concentrating on the entire work force or only a section of them. Then he should fix up timings for Observation. The important aspect among the other things, is what he should observe, for example, production environment, relationship between supervisor and workers, or relations among workers or anything. This enables the researcher to have a clear understanding about the problem, methodology and the necessary training for initiation of the project.
2. **Entry into the study environment:** The second step is entering the study environment. If the study is related to a governmental establishment, the permission of the appropriate authority may be necessary. If the study is related to a local group like the village panchayat, a letter from the proper channels should be supplemented with the approval of the key persons to gain entry into the study group. After gaining entry into the group, the observer should identify his role either as a participant observer or non-participant observer etc. He should also develop normal relationship with the group (i.e., the establishment of rapport). Then only the observer will become acceptable to the group. He should impress upon his informants about the confidentiality of their identification in the study.
3. **Initial interactions:** The researcher should establish preliminary contact with situation and initial interaction with the respondents. The researcher is required to use his ingenuity in mixing and interacting with the people.
4. **Observation and recording:** Observation normally does not pose a problem once rapport has been established. But recording the Observation poses a problem. The researcher should take utmost care in order not to disturb respondent's original or true behaviour. The researcher may use good mechanical devices to improve the recording facility and accuracy. The researcher should take care to record the events in sequence and see that is does not miss any important stage in a sequence in the whole process. Further he should verify the creditability of statements of respondents and accordingly classify the data even when he is recording the same.

5. **Termination of field work:** This last step involves not only the termination of research work on hand but also the termination of emotional relationships, if any, developed during the study. There should be no bias and distortion in the analysis and interpretation of data.

Aids in Observation Process

The use of tools like diaries, field notes, maps, checklists, cameras, audio and video tape recorders etc., may enhance precision to the Observation process. Let us discuss these aids briefly:

Diaries: The researcher after observing the situation can keep a record of each event. This may take the form of a diary. If carefully written, these things give a fair and sufficiently long account of the situation.

Field notes: An observer must record detailed notes of everything he observes. Distortion, which will hinder the progress of the work, must be avoided.

Maps: The utility of the map is not limited merely to the graphic portrayal of facts.

Maps are often indispensable in locating problem, verifying hypothesis, analyzing data and discovering hidden facts and relationships. The social base maps showing the relation of hypographical aspects of a community to its social organization will call for further study and Observation which probably would have never come to light otherwise.

Analogy: In analyzing a social institution or social relationship and in answering questions like how does someone become an embezzler? Analogies are particularly useful.

Checklist: It is one of the most basic structural methods of Observation. This device is often used in making Observation to ensure that an observer looks for every bit of evidence that he has previously determined as essential. It should be prepared in advance of the Observation but should include blank space for recording phenomena that were not anticipated in the formulation of the problem. There are two types of checklists-static and action.

In the static checklist such information as sex, race or age may be recorded together with the characteristics of environment. Action checklist are used to record actual behaviour. This technique is particularly appropriate for behaviour which has a limited number of alternatives. The investigator simply tallies whether the behaviour has occurred or not.

Sociometric scales: These were used in the measurement of social process of adjustment etc. These are regarded as tools or instruments of Observation with the same function as the physician's stethoscope or thermometer. The unique value of these scales is the increased clarity of the picture as compared to subjective judgements.

Sociometric measure is a measure of assessing the attraction and repulsions within a given group. Sociometric self-rating, scaling methods, group preferences, records, multi-relational sociometric survey etc., are some measures of sociometry.

Mechanical devices: Scientific instruments like microscope are used by the researchers in physical and natural sciences. In social science research, scholars take the help of devices like camera, tape recorder, video to record their observation and data. These devices help the researcher to present accurately a mass of detail in a concise and effective form.

TYPES OF OBSERVATION (CHOICE OF OBSERVATION TECHNIQUES)

Natural Vs. Contrived Observation

Natural Observation occurs when we observe behaviour as it is taking place in a normal setting, e.g., watching children while they select toys. In this type of Observation no attempt is made to manipulate the field of study or behaviour of the observed. These studies help the store managers to improve their collection of a particular variety. When researchers rely on natural direct observation, they frequently find themselves wasting a great deal of time while they wait for the desired event to happen. To reduce this problem Observation may be made efficiently. For example, in an actual study utilizing contrived observation, an uncombed and unshaven observer dressed in old clothes entered a departmental stores, then observed how many minutes it took before a sales person arrived to wait on him. The average was nearly 10 minutes. However, when the same individual was dressed in a sports coat and slacks he had the good fortune to be waited on in an average of just 5 minutes, a significant reduction. This enabled the researcher to conclude that the attentiveness of sales person is a function of customer dress.

Participant Observation (P.O)

When the observer participates with the activities of the group under study, it is known as P.O. The researcher mingles with the group and actively shares his activities with the life of the group on whom he is observing. Thus, a participant observer makes himself a part of the group under study. He freely mixes with social activities of the group. The purpose of critical study is concealed under the desire to learn folklores and more, customs and traditions.

Merits of Participant Observation: The observer can obtain more hidden aspects, significant and symbolic factors which are not easily exposed to others. He can gain more insight into understanding the group's social, economic, and political life. He can gather more information.

The observer should desist from acquiring any special status in the group. The moment he becomes emotionally involved, he may acquire bias and loose his identity as an observer and may not be in a position to do justice to the investigation.

Non-participant Observation (NPO)

When the observer does not actually participate in the activities of the group, but simply observes them from a distance, it is known as a N.P.O. Purely NPO is extremely difficult. However, being a stranger, the observer is less involved emotionally. He can maintain his own status as a researcher and it will help to maintain objectivity and impartiality.

An N.P.O. in practice is only a quasi-participant observation.

Controlled Observation (C.O.)

When observation takes place according to definite prearranged plans, involving experimental procedure, it is called controlled observation. This method affords greater precision and objective and can be repeatedly observed under identical conditions. The main purpose of a C.O. is to check any bias due to faulty perception, inaccurate data, and influence of outside factors on the particular incident.

Generally, controlled observation takes place in various experiments that are carried out in a laboratory or under controlled conditions.

The control exercised in the Observation is of two types:

(i) Control over the phenomena and

(ii) Control over the observation.

In the first type, the phenomena is put to laboratory type test under guided conditions. Such experiment was made to study the effect of lighting upon production. Various kinds of work studies come under this type. The study of the behaviour of children and infants also come under this type.

Control Over the Observation: When the phenomena under study can not be subjected to guided experiment, the researcher tries to control and guide his own perception and thus, to avoid any bias due to faulty observation. Following kinds of control devices are generally used for this purpose:

1. Detailed Observation plan,
2. Use of schedules,
3. Use of mechanical appliances,
4. Use of sociometric scales,
5. Use of hypothesis,
6. Team Observation, and
7. Use of control groups.

Non-controlled Observation

If the observation takes place in the natural setting, it may be termed as uncontrolled observation. No attempt is made to use any instruments, i.e., the mechanical aids are not used and the data are collected without standardizing procedure and without resorting to a random sample. When the Observation is made in the natural surroundings and the activities are performed in their usual course without being guided by any external force, it is non-controlled observation. The major aim is to get a spontaneous picture of life and persons. This type is not very reliable. However, most of the social phenomena have to be observed in an uncontrolled way.

Direct Observation (DO)

Under DO, actual behaviour, verbal or non-verbal, is observed first hand. For instance, to study student behaviour in a particular situation, you may just go and watch them while they are behaving in that situation.

Indirect Observation (IO)

Under this, results or physical traces of behaviour are observed. For example, from the traces the students have left, or the way the chairs are arranged or disarranged or from other scenes, you can guess how they would have behaved in that particular situation.

Overt and Covert Observation

In Overt Observation, those being observed are aware of the investigator's presence and intension. In Covert Observation, the investigator's presence is hidden or undisclosed or his or her intensions are disguised.

Structured and Unstructured Observation

If the observation is characterized by a careful definition of the units to be observed, standardardised conditions of observation and the selection of pertinent data of observation, it is called as structured observation (S.O). In S.O. the investigator looks for and systematically records the incidence of specific behaviours (incidents). This method is considered appropriate in descriptive studies. Unstructured observation is considered appropriate in exploratory research work. When no careful definitions and conditions are entertained, information is gathered in natural settings. It is called as unstructured observation (U.S.). In U.S., all behaviours are considered relevant at first and recorded, but later on, upon reflection the investigator will distinguish between the important and trivial behaviour.

Objectives of Observation

- Studying collective behaviour and complex social situations.
- Following up of individual units composing the situations.
- Understanding the whole and the parts in their interrelations.
- Getting out of the way the details of the situations.

Reliability and Success of Observation

(i) The observed problem must be formulated very clearly and precisely,

(ii) The observer must develop a free and open mind,

(iii) Only vital elements should be considered,

(iv) Suitable technique and tools should be used, and

(v) The quality of the observer should be high.

IMPORTANCE OF OBSERVATION

- It is the simplest and most non-technical method.
- It is one of the main sources of formulating hypothesis.
- Observation, at times, affords greater accuracy than other methods.
- The data collected through Observation is more convincing than otherwise. It is most important in testing the validity of the hypothesis framed.
- It is a common method for all sciences. It helps to study the subject in depth.
- It helps in the free flow of information.
- It is possible to record behaviour as it occurs.
- It is a very useful technique of studying various activities and characteristics of infants and children.

- The researcher is able to record natural behaviour of the group.
- He can collect a wide range of information.
- It is an useful method of doing research in delicate areas.
- It is less expensive.

PLANNING AND EXECUTION OF OBSERVATION

1. The observer must have a sound background of theory and knowledge in the area of his study.
2. The researcher must carefully select and define clearly and preciously the activities to be observed.
3. The next important aspect is formulation of testable hypothesis.
4. The researcher must decide the size of units to be observed.
5. He must decide the type of Observation technique to be used.
6. He must determine the period to be observed.
7. He should select appropriate aids and mechanical devices to be employed.
8. The researcher must also decide the number of observers needed.
9. He must arrange for expert training to the observers.
10. He must arrange for preliminary Observation.
11. He must arrange for proper recording of data.
12. After data have been collected, he has to pay full attention to their analysis and interpretation.

LIMITATIONS

1. All occurrences may not be open to Observation.
2. Personal bias distorts the Observation.
3. Systematic and preplanned Observation is very difficult.
4. Natural factors such as weather conditions may affect the observational task.
5. There are difficulties in sampling.
6. Faulty perception.
7. The researcher's interpretation is mostly impressionistic.
8. Some historical events are not open to direct observation.
9. The information gathered may be in tune with the whims and fancies of the observer.
10. This method is useful only in the case of relatively small group or system.

CHAPTER 8

Report Writing

Report writing is a basic task of the researcher because no research can be completed without its report. It is the end product of a research activity. Research reporting is the oral or written presentation of evidence (i.e., the findings of the study). Research report writing is culmination of the research investigation. Reporting is the end product of a research activity. It is a highly skilled work. Report writing is the final stage of the research. Report writing is a technical activity which requires considerable thought, effort, patience and skill. In fact, a report is not a complete description of what has been actually done during the period of investigation, but it is only a brief statement of significant facts that are necessary for understanding the generalization drawn by the researcher. In report writing there arises several problems regarding the language vocabulary, style etc.

NEED FOR REPORT (OBJECTIVES OF REPORT WRITING)

A researcher needs to report his results on following reasons:

1. **Search for knowledge:** The purpose of research is to search for knowledge. A research scholar has an obligation to report to the community as to what emerged in his search. This gives rise to the necessity of communicating one's own results and thoughts to the people and fellow scientists.
2. **Evolution of theory:** A research report is needed to evolve a theory or principle. It is only after a thorough discussion a principle or a theory is evolved.

3. **Exchange of ideas:** Reporting is the process through which a basic ground is prepared for the exchange of ideas or thoughts. Unless a scientist reports in a journal or at a conference the results of his study, there will not be any opportunity for others to accept or reject his proposition.
4. **To make specific recommendations:** Reporting helps the researcher to make specific recommendations for a course of action.
5. **To reveal ability:** The research ability of the candidate is revealed through the final report he presents.
6. **Useful for all:** A research report is highly useful for policy formulators, practitioners, the general public and others.
7. To highlight the order of presentation in business research.
8. To understand the dynamics of drawing inferences and generalization in business.
9. To illustrate different types of report writing and the contents to be followed in reports.

TYPES OF REPORTS

A preliminary classification of reports is into two types, namely, oral and written reports.

ORAL REPORT

What goes on in seminars, conferences, symposia etc., is mainly oral presentation. The merit of this approach lies in the fact that it provides an opportunity for give and take decisions which generally lead to a better understanding of the findings and their implication.

At seminars, the research scholars are allowed to present an oral report. Viva voce is an, e.g., for this type of report. But the main demerit of this sort of presentation is the lack of any permanent record concerning the research details. The findings may fade away from people's memory even before an action is taken. Oral presentation is effective when supplemented by various visual devices like slides and charts.

WRITTEN REPORT

Presentation of information or results in writing requires many qualities and a great deal of effort by the researcher. Utmost attention should be paid for writing the research report.

Written report themselves are of different types. In the context of reporting to management of a company, reports are classified as

1. External and internal reports,

2. Routine and special reports, and
3. Operating report.

In addition, the reporting may be

1. Lower level reporting,
2. Middle level reporting, and
3. Top level reporting.

On the basis of the people to whom the report is meant, written report may be

1. Popular report,
2. Report for the administrator, and
3. Technical report.

1. Popular report: This is the report meant to be read by general public or layman. It should present broad facts, findings, and recommendations. It must be interesting, simple and lucid. It must avoid all technical jargons and details as to the method of investigation. For example, in a study of Indian economy, the layman is interested in how the economy is performing in broad terms and what is going to happen to their standard of living. They are not generally interested in such details as to the capital – output ratio etc.

2. Report for administrator: Many of the business reports are of this type. They may be submitted to any level. These reports are prepared for a specific purpose. These reports should neither be too general nor too technical. It may contain some technical aspects but on the whole simple and direct.

3. Technical report: A technical report is written by an expert to be read by another expert. In this sense, a thesis is a technical report intended to be read by another researcher. Not only thesis, but even a monograph, and a journal article are technical aspects both in the sampling methods and subject matter. In a technical report conceptual and analytical frame work and sample design are adequately explained. A technical report is written for the fellow researcher and therefore, should be organized on a different footing altogether. The four distinguishing facts of technical reports are:

1. The problem and its nature,
2. The method and its scientific accuracy,
3. The data and their dependability, and
4. The logical relationship of the data and the interpretation.

These facts have to be presented logically and sequentially with simplicity, clarity and brievity. A general outline of a technical report can be as follows:

1. Summary of results (in two or three pages).
2. Nature of the study (and objectivity of study, formulations of the problem, hypothesis, type of analysis etc.).
3. Methods employed.
4. Data (primary and secondary data).
5. Main body of the report (in several chapters).
6. Analysis of data and presentation of findings (tables, charts etc.).

The **time-sequence pattern of report writing** (or step-by step presentation) is a way of presenting the events in an operation frequently following one another at a point of time. It is adapted to report on manufacturing operations.

The **inductive pattern of report writing** is one of the oldest patterns of presenting one's thoughts. This type of report goes from the specific to general recommendations, summary, conclusions, etc.

The deductive pattern of report writing (also known as the executive report, the management report, or the action-getting report) is the pattern of presentation that goes from the general to the specific (i.e., from the more important to the less important). It is the most accepted type of report writing in the business world.

A project report is the report of a project undertaken by an individual or a group of individuals or any functional area or any aspect or segment of any functional area of the business, industry, or society. It is a detailed report written with a specific purpose in mind.

A business report or memorandum may be defined as a simple business communication from one departmental head to another, one functional area to another, or from top to bottom in the organizational structure on any specific aspect of day-to-day business activity. It is a brief observational report that assists one in arriving at a business decision.

A dissertation is a detailed report on the subject of the study that was undertaken. This is a document submitted for the acquisition of a higher degree from a university.

A thesis, too, is a detailed dissertation, which maintains a valuable proposition or hypothesis, written on the basis of a detailed research. Thesis is used for academic purpose.

A commission's enquiry report is a detailed report prepared by a commission appointed for the specific purpose of conducting a detailed study of any matter of dispute or of anything which requires a greater insight so that it may facilitate a future course of action. It is an expert opinion.

Essentials of a good report: (principles in report writing or principles of effective thesis writing)

1. **Clarity and coherence:** Clarity is the first essential requirement of a good research report. The researcher should be first clear in his writing. Research report writing is a reasoning process and without clarity of thought, there would not be clarity in writing.
2. **Writing correctly:** A research report should be written correctly. Incorrect writing is frequently ambiguous, sometimes quite misleading and usually difficult to understand. To write correctly, one has to know grammar. Incorrect writing leaves a poor opinion about the researcher and his work. The researcher should have a good command over the language. But he should not use complex high sounding language at the cost of clarity. He should always remember that he is writing scientific report and not a magazine article.
3. **Brievity:** The researcher should take care of the economy of words and concentration of ideas. Repetition and superfluousness will obstruct the lucidity of the report and will interfere with precision and clarity.
4. **Objectivity:** The report should be written in an unbiased manner objectivity of the report should be fortified by facts.
5. **Styled to the reader's taste:** A good report is one that is written in style that the audience can follow. The style should suit the focus group. It should convince the audience the truth and the ideas presented in the report.
6. **Readability:** Chistine Browning found the following seven ways of defining readability:
   (i) Readability is the absence if jargon and slang.
   (ii) Readability is never having to read twice.
   (iii) Readability is consistent terminology.
   (iv) Readability is short paragraph.
   (v) Readability is short sentences.
   (vi) Readability is continuity.
   (vii) Readability is clarity.
7. **Effective (neat) arrangement:** Proper organization of the report is the important ingredient in the whole process. Simply to know that a report has an introduction, body, and conclusion is of little use. The real problem is to decide where to begin and what to say next. This deals with the different parts of a report. It refers to the arrangement of ideas in a logical and coherent manner.

8. **Planning and organizing:** Planning and organizing the study materials form the basis of preparing the research report. A well conceived planning and organizing the report facilitates report writing with proper emphasis to different aspects.
9. **Interest and appeal:** A researcher should not write on anything that does not interest him and that which does not appeal to him.
10. **Primarily a craft:** Thesis writing is primarily a craft that should be mastered by a researcher.
11. **Fitfull and well communication:** One of the rules governing effective thesis writing is that every researcher must realize that his single aim should be to communicate to the readers fitfully and well.
12. **Judicious selection of materials:** There must be a judicious selection of the materials to convey and the means with which to convey thesis, i.e., good writing is never accidental.
13. **Avoid personal opinion:** An effective thesis writer should avoid using phrases of personal opinion such as it appears to me, it seems to us, I am sure, to quote a few, etc.
14. **Things to remember:** The researcher should remember
    (i) Not to use clinches.
    (ii) Not to use sentence in fragments.
    (iii) Not to resort to figurative language too often.
    (iv) Not to be ambiguous.
    (v) Not to repeat the same idea.
    (vi) Not to say of a thing of which be is not clear.
15. **Concentration on central idea:** The researcher must concentrate on the central idea of his dissertation and relate every other aspects to it.
16. **Faith in his capacities:** The researcher must have faith in his capacities and he must write with a sense of purpose and conviction.
17. **Acknowledgement:** Another proper principle of writing is not to plagiarize. Therefore, whatever materials used to support or refute an argument, it must be acknowledged with due credit being given to the authors of such evidence.
18. The other principle of good thesis writing is that there must be an effective introduction, sound body – part of the thesis and a satisfactory summation.

PROBLEMS IN REPORT WRITING

The following problems are encountered by the researcher in writing a research report:

1. **The problem of communication:** The problem of communication is the basic problem of report writing. The findings of the study generally constitute technical knowledge which may not be easy for the lay man to understand. Hence, the researcher has to keep in mind the fact that the report is not meant only for technical hands or for those possess technical knowledge while writing the report.
2. **Problem of objectivity:** In social research, objectivity is a guiding factor. The presentation of the data collected should be very objective. It means that the report should be free from prejudices and bias. This is of much importance especially while writing report in social science.
3. **Problems of expressing bitter truth and unpleasant facts:** It is necessary for the researcher to include in his report even those facts which are quite bitter and unpleasant for certain group of people. Unless the conclusions that are based on entire data collected are given in the report, the report shall be loop-sided. In presentation of bitter facts and unpleasant truths, the researcher has to do tight rope-walking. It means that he has to present these facts in a manner which is not offending the feelings of a particular group of peoples.

GUIDELINES FOR REPORT WRITING

While writing a research report the following guidelines are to be followed:

Length of Report

While determining the report one should keep in mind the fact that it should be reasonably long enough to cover the subject but short enough to maintain interest.

Attractive Style

While writing a research report, one has to adopt his style of communicating the results. Style includes the art of selecting and arranging words to communicate a message in a way appropriate to the needs of the reader. It is, in fact, this style which distinguishes a typical report.

Style is important for many reasons. Firstly, it helps to clarify one's own thinking and secondly, it helps to convey one's own thoughts clearly to an audience or readers. Style matters much especially in the case of business research because the audience is made up of specialists who are intelligent task-oriented, busy and impatient.

Avoidance of Technical Terms

The report should avoid the use of abstract terminology and technical jargons as far as possible. The report should be able to convey the matter as simply as possible. It must be written in an objective style and in simple language.

Ready Availability of Findings

Readers are often interested in acquiring a quick knowledge of main findings and as such the report must provide a ready availability of the findings. For this purpose, charts, diagrams and statistical tables may be used for the various results in the main report in addition to the summary of main findings.

THE LAYOUT OF THE REPORT

The layout of the report should be well throughout and must be appropriate and in accordance with the objectives of the research problem.

Grammatical Accuracy

The reports should be free from grammatical mistakes. They must be prepared strictly in accordance with the techniques of composition of report writing such as the use of quotations, foot notes, documentation, proper punctuation and use of abbreviations in the foot notes and the like.

Logical Analysis

The report must present the logical analysis of the subject matter. It must reflect a structure wherein the different pieces of analysis relating to the research problem fit well.

Originality

A research report should demonstrate clearly the originality of the researcher. It should necessarily constitute an attempt to solve some intellectual problem. It must contribute to the solution of a problem and must add to the store of knowledge.

Policy Implications

The report must state, towards the end the policy implications relating the problem under consideration. It is usually considered desirable if the report makes a forecast of the probable feature of the subject concerned and indicates the kinds of research that could be taken up by the future researchers.

Objective of the Study

The research report should state clearly in the beginning such things as objectives of the study, nature of the problem, the methods employed and techniques of analysis in the form of introduction.

Appendices

The report must contain list of appendices in respect of those technical data at the end. The appendices may contain the methodology described in technical jargon for the fellow researchers and experts. They may contain raw data and documents not readily accessible. The following books provide useful guidelines for thesis writing:

Albaugh, R.W.: Thesis Writing; A Guide to Scholarly Style, 1955, Patterson, New Jersey, Littlefield, Adams.

Campbell, W.C.: Form and Style in Thesis Writing, 1956, Houghton Mifflin, Cambridge, Mass, the U.S.A.

Anderson and others: Thesis and Assignment Writing 1970, Wiley Eastern (P) Ltd., New Delhi.

Bibliography

Bibliography is the descriptive list of books. It is a list of all sources that the writer has consulted while doing research. It is the systematic preparation of a list of books. It is also the technique of systematically producing descriptive lists of written or published records. It is a list of books or writings of one author or about one subject. It is the study of books. It is about the knowledge of books with regard to authors, subjects, edition and history. A book containing a descriptive list of books may be known as bibliography. It is a study of the authorship, editions etc. of books.

The Association of Indian Universities (AIU) had started preparing bibliography of these is accepted by Indian Universities for the award of Ph.D, early in 1935 itself. Since 1978, the AIU has been publishing bibliographies every year.

The term reference is used almost synonymously to the other terms such as work cited, source consulted and select bibliography. The purpose is to provide an index of the materials consulted for thesis writing. Every book, article, thesis, document or manuscript which has been read or examined and cited should be included in the select bibliography. However, there are no absolute rules on referencing. The system adopted is influenced by the system of foot-noting used in the body of the thesis, the requirement of the institutions conferring the degree.

Bibliography should contain essential information such as: (a) the author or authors, (b) the title of publication, (c) Publisher, and (d) the year of publication.

In case of a journal-article, additional information regarding the name of the journal, volume, number, month and year of publication and pages become relevant. However, in case of a journal-article, the place of publication is not included. The usual style of citing reference is given below: Mustafa. A, Case Study Methods – Theory and Practice, Atlantic Publishers, ISBN 978-81-269-1006-9, 2008, p/pp. .... .

Tips for Writing Bibliography

(i) Alphabetize the author's name or by first main word in article or book.

(ii) List only those sources you actually used in your thesis.

(iii) Your bibliography comes at the very end of your thesis.

(iv) If your list contains more than one book by the same author, after the first entry in his name, substitute a line followed by a period instead of repeating the name. For example:

Hicks, J.R.: Value and Capital, 2nd ed. (London: Oxford, 1946) ________ A Revision of Demand Theory (London: Oxford, 1956)

(v) Do not use numbers in bibliography listings.

(vi) Use a hanging bibliography form. Indent five spaces from second line.

Types of Bibliographies

Historical Bibliographies: This traces the various methods of book production printing processes, and the embellishments that are employed.

Analytical Bibliographies: They analyze the structure of the book and present an accurate description of the form and content of the book listed.

Systematic Bibliography: It methodically concerns itself with the preparation of the list of books.

Critical Bibliography: It embraces the methods adopted by the analytical and historical types.

Annotated Bibliography: Contains a brief statement explaining the significance of each entry.

Preliminary Bibliography and Final Bibliography (PB & FB): Both are of two parts viz., the primary source which is prepared chronologically and the secondary source which is classified and listed alphabetically. While PB lists the books and articles, primary and secondary, that are extended on the chosen subject, the FB should contain the particulars of the books and articles that have been referred to by the scholar. PB refers to list of books and articles referred to at the preliminary stage of research and the FB refers to the final solid list of books referred to by the scholars at the final stage of research.

Units of bibliography entry: The first unit concerns itself with the name of the author or names of authors. The second unit deals with the title of the journal, article or the critical essay in an anthology or title of the books. The third unit presents the facts of publication namely the place of publication, the publisher's name.

Bibliography is the list of books, journals and other works which were consulted while carrying out the research work. Bibliography should be arranged alphabetically and may be divided into two portions. The first portion may contain the names of books and pamphlets and the second portion may contain the name of magazines and newspaper article. When a researcher begins to consult a new source, he should make out a source or bibliography card for it. Models of bibliography or source cards:

For a book by one or two authors:

Call number	:	ISBN 978-81-8054-449-5 | Source Card No.
Author	:	A. Mustafa
Title	:	Research Methodology
Publication	:	A.I.T.B.S. Publishers, India
Information	:	Delhi – 110051

It is essential to keep a separate, complete and accurate card record of each source of information in the above manner, for a newspaper article, for an encyclopaedia and for a magazine article etc., consulted.

A list of references used for the purpose of writing the research report should be prepared and appended to the research report.

With reference to quotations, remember the following:

(i) Use quotation marks if the note is a direct quotation.

(ii) If you omit words from the quotation, indicate the omission with eclipses marks (four periods thus. ...)

(iii) Quote accurately. Even if an error exists in the text, copy it and follow it with (S/C), which means 'thus in the original'.

A short quotation–consisting of fewer than five lines–should be in quotation marks and combined smoothly as part of your own sentence; for example: A long quotation consisting of more than one sentence should be set off from the text of the paper by the following procedures:

(A) Double space above and below the quotation.

(B) Single space the quoted material.

(C) Indent the quoted an additional five spaces on both sides.

(D) Do not use quotation marks; the single spacing and extra indentation are sufficient to indicate that the passage is in quotation.

Note Card: The researcher should write his notes on uniform cards (3″ × 5″ or 4″ × 6″ following the instructions given below:

(i) Write on one side of the card only.

(ii) Only one topic and one source should be on each card.

(iii) Include in upper left hand corner, the topic of the one specific subject treated on that card, for identification of source, note the bibliography card number in right hand corner, notes on material intended for use in the centre and the pages where this material is found in the left margin.

(iv) If you wish to quote material from a source, copy it accurately and completely and enclose it in quotation marks.

(v) Otherwise, take notes in your own words as briefly as possible. Let the notes be fair summaries of the material read. Use abbreviation and incomplete sentences so long as they would be intelligible to you later on.

(vi) Do not take down the obvious, easily remembered well-known or general facts. Record only facts which are new to you or stated in an unusual way.

(vii) Include all the details needed for footnotes and bibliography.

(viii) If you find it necessary to continue your notes start a new card with correct topic information. Each card should be complete in itself.

The research report must also give the sources consulted for data collection analysis. The bibliography is typed at the end of the main body of the research report. The purpose of the bibliography is to identify the whole work. The references used are arranged in alphabetical order. It may be under different headings such as books, journals, reports, newspapers, public documents and miscellaneous.

INDEX

Index is also considered as an essential part of a good report. It must be prepared and appended at the end.

Limitations

The researcher must state clearly the various constraints and limitations faced by him while conducting the research study. This would help appreciate the reliability of the data collected, analyzed and inferences drawn.

Conclusions

The research scholar should develop his thesis by writing in a controlled fashion never succumbing to personal preferences and biased views. We should not indulge in personal attacks. In thesis writing, self-evident propositions should be avoided. Yet again, thesis writing should not be of a cataloguing kind. It should be all of these. Above all a thesis should not argue two propositions at random. In fact, a good thesis is built on a sound proposition that invites arguments.

STEPS IN REPORT WRITING

The usual steps involved in writing a research report are as follows:

Logical analysis of the subject matter

In this step, the development of the subject is considered. There are two ways by which a subject can be developed. This is (a) logically and (b) chronologically. Whereas the logical development is made on the basis of mental connections and associations, chronological development is done on the basis of time sequence.

(a) **Preparation of the final outline:** This constitutes the preparation of outline on the basis of which written works are to be constructed. This helps in logical organization of the material.

(b) **Preparation of rough draft:** After carrying out the logical analysis in the subject and preparing the final outline, the researcher then prepares a rough draft of his research study. In this draft details regarding the methodology adopted for data collection and analysis, limitations of the study and broad-findings and suggestions are given.

(c) **Revision of rough draft:** This constitutes re-writing and polishing the rough draft of the research study which has been already completed. This implies writing in a logical way and presenting in clear and coherent manner the results of the study. While revising the rough draft, the researcher should check the aspects of writing-grammar spelling and usage.

(d) **Preparation of Bibliography** (For details refer to page 181).

(e) **Writing the final draft:** This constitutes the last step in the process of writing the research project. The final draft should be written in concise and an objective style and in simple language avoiding strange expressions. Care must be taken by the researcher to avoid abstract terminology and technical jargons. The final draft must be interesting and should reflect the originality of the researcher.

MECHANICS OF REPORT WRITING

This explains the set of rules which govern the actual preparation of a research report. The following are the various aspects which are considered in writing of a research report.

Size and Physical Design

The manuscript should be written on unruled paper which is 8″ × 11″ in size. If it is written by hand, then, black or blue-black ink should be used a margin of at least 1′ and 1″ should be allowed on the left hand side and of at least an inch at the right hand side of the paper. There should also be 1 inch margin top and bottom. The paper should be neat and eligible.

Procedure

While writing a research report, the researcher should carefully take into consideration various types that are usually followed.

1. Layout

The layout of a research report should be determined keeping in mind the objective and the nature of the problem. A comprehensive layout of the research report should comprise:

(a) Preliminary pages

(b) Main text

(c) The end matter.

2. Treatment of Quotations

Quotations should be placed in quotation marks and double space forming an immediate part of the text. However, if a quotation is of a considerable length extending to four or five lines then it may be single spaced.

3. The Foot Notes

Foot notes are normally found at the foot of a page. Foot notes serve the purpose of identification of materials that are used in quotations in the report. They are meant for cross references, situation of authorities and sources, acknowledgement and explanation of a point of view. Generally, the use of foot notes in a research report goes to demonstrate the scholarship of the researcher. The foot notes should contain specific information derived from the bibliography cards. When one borrows an idea or the logic of an argument, one must acknowledge indebtedness in foot note. The foot notes include the source of information, the title of the source, exact page(s) of the source of reference, date of publication and publisher and place of publication. Following points are to be considered while using foot notes in a report.

- They are to be placed at the bottom of the page on which the relevant reference ends.

- They are to be shown separately from the textual material by a space of an inch and about 1 inch long.
- They are to be numbered consequently, usually beginning with one in each chapter separately.
- The number should be put slightly above the line, say, at the end of the quotation.
- They are to be typed in single space and to be divided from one another by double space.

Use a foot note to:

- Single space footnotes which require more than one line.
- Note that the author's first name or initials should be written first.
- Give credit for a direct quotation.
- If you find a quotation in one source that is got from another source, list both sources.
- Give credit for statistics, figures, definitions, illustrations or diagrammes.
- Give credit for an original or unusually interesting opinion or interpretation which you have put in your own words.
- Number foot notes consecutively throughout a chapter. Begin numbering afresh in the next chapter.
- The foot note number is placed in the text right after the statement like an exponent.
- Place number (again above the line without a period, i.e., a full stop) and its foot note at the bottom of the page. Indent the first line of each foot note and start the second line even with the left margin.
- If a source is repeated, you need only list last name of the author followed up by *op.cit.* and a page reference. If it is also the same page reference, use *loc.cit.* If a source is the same as the one immediately above, *ibid.*, with the page number, if different.

Examples of Footnotes: The first time a source is acknowledged:

The first time a particular source is acknowledged in a foot note. The source must be completely identified as in the following examples:

(i) For a book by one author:

A. Mustafa: Case Study Methods: Theory and Practice, Atlantic Publications, New Delhi, 2008.

G. Von Haberler, *Prosperity and Description* (Geneva, League of Nations, 1941), p. 85.

(ii) For a book with two authors:

Gerald M. Meir and Robert E. Baldwin, *Economic Development Theory, History and Policy* (New York, John Wiley and Sons Inc. 1957), p. 43.

(iii) For a book with no author's name:

Webster's Biological, p. 500.

(iv) For a book which is edited or a critical edition:

K.S. Sonachalam, Ed. *Theory of Economic Development*, Annamalai University, Annamalai Nagar, 1967, Dr. John D.K. Sundarsingh: Agriculture and Village Development, p. 142.

(v) For an Encyclopedia article:

Encyclopedia, Vol. VI, p. 456.

(vi) For a signed magazine article:

'Defence Expenditure After 1960', by B. Natarajan, *The Eastern Economist*, May 12, 1978, p. 936.

(vii) For an unsigned magazine article or an editorial:

'Cheap Loans and Rural Poor', The Hindu (May 26, 1977), p. 6.

(viii) For material from one source quoted in another:

Alexander Gerschenkron, "Economic Backwardness in Historical Perspective" in Bert F. Hoselitz, editor, *The Progress of Underdeveloped Areas* (University of Chicago Press, Chicago, 1952), p. 27-59, quoted by P.A. Samuelson in *Economics*, McGraw Hill Book Company, Inc. New York, 1958.

Examples of shortened form of foot notes for sources previously acknowledged:

1. For a book which has been cited in the immediately preceding foot note, *ibid*, p. 254.
2. When the work has been cited before but not in the immediately preceding foot-note the following forms are used:
   (i) For a book by one author when only one work by that author has been cited: Mary Joseph, "Alfred Nobel – A Life Story", p.4.
   (ii) Some authorities recommended the use of the expression op, cit. for the title that has already been referred to as Mary Joseph, op. cit. p.26.
3. When using more than one work by the same author, use a shorthand form of the title that has already been referred to. For example, if you are using three books by J.M. Keynes, use this form, Shakespearian Sonnets, p. 67.

Documentation Style

The documentary foot note references giving all the essential facts about the addition used shall be shown. The usual order which is followed for showing such a reference is as follows:

- Author's name followed by a comma,
- Title of work, to be shown in Italics,
- Name, Place and Date of Publication, and
- Page Numbers.

If the same work is sited again without any other work intervening, it may be indicated as Ibid followed by a comma and a page number. Where a single page is referred, it is indicated as p. However, where more than one page has been referred it shall be indicated as pp.

Punctuation and Abbreviations in Foot Notes

The first item after the number in the foot note is the author's name given in the normal signature order. This is followed by a comma. After the comma the title of the book is given: the article (such as the a, an etc.) is omitted and only the first word and only the proper words and adjectives are shown in letters, information concerning the edition is given next which is followed by the place of the publication, name of publisher and data of publication. Then follows the volume and page references.

Use of Statistics, Diagrams and Graphs

Generally, a judicious use of statistics in research reports is considered an important requirement. For it contributes in large measure towards the clarification and simplification of the materials and research results. Statistical data are usually presented in the form of tables, charts and diagrams. Such presentation needs to be self-explanatory and complete in all aspects.

The Final Draft

This constitutes the revising and re-writing of the rough draft of the report. The researcher should consider the grammatical correctness and logical arrangement of information in the report.

PREPARATION OF THE INDEX

The index serves as a good guide to the reader. This is given at the end of the report. This may be prepared both as subject index and as author index. Whereas the subject index gives the names of subject topics along with the page number on which they have been discussed in the report, the author index gives similar information regarding the names of authors. The index should always be arranged in the alphabetical order.

FORMAT OF THE RESEARCH REPORT

The following outline presents the usual sequence of various section of the Report:

A. Preliminary Section

- Title page
- Approval sheet
- Acknowledgement
- Preface (Foreword)
- Table of contents
- List of tables
- List of figures.

B. Main Body of the Report

(i) Introduction
- Significance of the problem
- Statement of the problem
- Purpose of the study
- Assumptions and delimitations
- Definition of important terms
- Statement of hypotheses
- Assumptions underlying the hypotheses

(ii) Review of literature (analysis of previous research).

(iii) Design of the study
- Procedures used
- Methods of gathering data
- Description of data gathering instruments

(iv) Presentation and analysis of data
- Text
- Tables
- Figures.

(v) Summary and conclusions
   - Brief restatement of problem and procedures
   - Description of procedures used
   - Principal findings and conclusions
   - Recommendations for further research.

C. Reference Section
- Bibliography
- Appendix
- Index.

Methods of Collecting Primary Data

They are information collected by the researcher for the purposes of the project immediately at hand.

By observation: This method implies the collection of information by way of investigator's own observation. The information obtained relates to the current behaviour of the respondents. This method is expensive. Moreover, the information is very limited. Hence, this method is not suitable for large sample inquiry.

Through personal interview: Here, the investigator gets answer to a set of questions through personal interview. The success of this investigation depends on the ability of the interviewer.

Through telephone interview: The investigator contacts the respondents on telephone. This method is not widely used. But it is used in industrial surveys in developing regions.

By mailing of questionnaires: This method is quite popular in case of big enquiries. A questionnaire is sent by post to the persons concerned with a request to answer the question and return the questionnaire. Before applying this method, usually a pilot study for testing the questionnaire is conducted.

Through schedules: The trained enumerators go to the respondents with schedules containing questions. Data are collected by filling up the schedules by enumerators on the basis of replies given by respondents.

Secondary data: May be complied from (i) published sources, (ii) unpublished sources. The researcher, adopting the analytical method, depends entirely on secondary data. Sources may also be classified as (i) internal and (ii) external. Internal sources of data represents the data that are already available with the research organization or company. All that is available with outside organizations falls into external source. The external source again can be divided into (a) personal source and (b) public source.

The major **sources of secondary data.** They refer to the information that have been collected by someone other than a researcher for purposes other than those involved in the research project at hand.

(1) Printed books, papers, literature and magazine,
(2) Documents,
(3) Remains,
(4) Materials of cultural history and of analytical history,
(5) Diaries,
(6) Memories,
(7) Confessions,
(8) Sacred National Archieves, and the Record Offices at the State level,
(9) Autobiographies,
(10) Diplomatic agreements,
(11) Statistical materials,
(12) Supressed inventions,
(13) Personal letters,
(14) Personal accounts,
(15) Personal sources of authentic observers and witness,
(16) Artistic materials,
(17) Official or public sector bodies which, in their turn, may be classified into: (i) Ministries, Departments, (ii) Special agencies, e.g., NSSO, CSO, RBI, ICAR, Labour Bureau, Ministry of Labour and Office of the Registrar-General and Census Commissioner.
(18) Publications of ILO, IMF, WHO etc.
(19) Central and State Govt., published and unpublished reports. Such as Mandal Commission Report,
(20) Semiofficial publications,
(21) Publication of private bodies such as Chamber of Commerce,
(22) Publications of research organizations,
(23) Annual reports of public sector organizations,
(24) Letters,
(25) Non-official or private agencies which include (i) the Chambers of Commerce and Industry, Research Institutions, FICCI, etc., (ii) Independent institutions like the Institute of Economic Growth, NCAER, Madras. Institute of Applied Manpower Research etc., (iii) Universities, IIT etc., and (iv) Contemporaneous literature comprises both historical and current, e.g.,

Megasthenese Indica, Persian Chronicles, Arthasastra, year books, Samuel Pepys and Ananda Rangapillai's diary, etc.

The secondary data provide the much needed background information of various problems in different areas of study, reveal to the researcher the various problems already done in specific fields and help to avoid duplication of work. The researcher should select any one or a combination of two or more sources for collecting data. He has to take into consideration the nature of investigation, objective and scope of the inquiry, financial resources, available time, desired degree of accuracy and status of the investigator. Much depends upon the ability and experience of the researcher. Here, common sense is the chief requisite and experience is the chief teacher.

MAILED QUESTIONNAIRE

A questionnaire is a tool or device for securing answers to the set of questions by the respondent who fills in the form of questionnaire himself. A **schedule** is a list of questions, which helps to collect data from the field. This is generally filled in by the enumerator or the researcher or the interviewer himself. Mail order questionnaire is the most popular method. It contains many questions pertaining to the field of inquiry and provides space for answers. The questionnaire attempts to elicit opinions on various problems. Sometimes the questionnaire is filled by the enumerator or the interviewer in which case it is known as schedule. The schedules are those used in personal interviews whereas questionnaires are the forms distributed through mail. The questionnaire/schedule is an indispensable tool in social science research. The Questionnaire is a data collection instrument to be filled out by an informant. The questionnaire like the schedule is designed to collect data from large, diverse and widely scattered groups of people. The Questionnaire is generally sent through the mail to informants to be answered as specified in a covering letter. The schedule, on the other hand, is generally filled out by the researcher/ enumerator, who can interpret the questions when necessary. Webster defines a schedule as a formal list, a catalogue or inventory and it may be added that it is a counting device, used in formal and standard inquiries. The sole purpose is aiding in the collection of quantitative cross-sectional data. For the regular programme of the Bureau of the Census (U.S.A.), the usual practice is to call the collection forms, and schedules; but for special studies-conducted for other governmental agencies or for non-profit research organizations–the forms are generally referred to as Qustionnaires. They are beneficial and supplementary and extending devices in observation, in interviews and in evaluating personal behaviour and social situations. They also aid in standardizing and objectifying observations and interviews and finally they are useful devices for isolating one element at a time and thus intensifying observation of it.

Types of Schedules

1. **Observation Schedules or Forms:** (One observer or several may be employed to secure uniformly systematic data in an observation study.
2. **Document Schedules:** They are used for recording data obtained from documents, case histories and other materials).
3. **Institutional Survey Forms or Evaluation Schedules:** Schedules of this type are used to visualize the problems faced by or inherent in a given type of institution.
4. **Structured Questionnaires** are those which pose definite, concrete and pre-designed questions, that is, they are prepared in advance and not constructed on the spot during the question period (Pauline V. Young). Most questionnaire studies made in marketing research are of the structured type. The structured Questionnaire may be further categorized into two: (a) **Closed form and (b) Open End Questionnaire:** The open end Questionnaire is one in which the respondents has full choice of using his own style and diction of language, expression, length and perception. The respondents is not restricted in his replies to the question and his answers may be free and spontaneous. A closed-form Questionnaire is one in which questions are set in such manner that it leaves only a few alternatives answers. It may be of two types:

(i) **Yes-No, Right-wrong or True-False**

(ii) **Multiple-Choice Form** three or more suggested answers. The **Unstructured Questionnaire** contains a set of questions which are not structured in advance and which may be adjusted according to the needs of question period. It gives sufficient scope for a variety of answers. It is used mainly for conducting interviews. This type of questioning secures more information from the respondents who is not kept in the strait jacket of a set list of questions. This flexibility on part of the interviewer is a major advantage of the method, but it is also a major weakness. Since each interviewer handles each interview differently, it is difficult to compare results. Average and percentage cannot be compared with validity.

Disguised methods are designed, so that the respondents do not know what the objective of the study is. Such disguised methods may also be unstructured. Projective techniques are an example of this type.

The pictorial questionnaire is also used in rural areas for collection of data (from children or illiterate persons).

Questionnaire may be either **Codified Questionnaire or Uncodified Questionnaire:** Data obtained in structured, non-disguised studies are easier to tabulate and interpret than data gathered in other ways. Structured non-disguised studies can be handled by telephone, mail or personal interview.

Structured, Disguised Questionnaire: It has the advantage of disguise, primarily that respondents do not know what is being measured and hence are not biased in their answers.

Non-structured, Non-disguised Questionnaire: No formal questionnaire is used in this type. Instead of approaching respondents with a fixed list of questions, the interviewer attempts to get respondents to talk freely about the subject of interest. By doing so, the interviewer hopes to put respondents at ease and encourages them to express any idea which they have on the subject. The investigator gets more information from the respondent who is not kept in the strait jacket of a set list of questions.

Non-structured, Disguised Questionnaire: The clinical psychologists have developed disguised methods of gathering information. Disguised methods are designed so that the respondents do not know what the objective of the study is. Such disguised methods may also be unstructured. Projective techniques are an example of this type. Various projective techniques are used but the most common are word association, sentence compilation and story telling. When individuals describe a situation, they are actually describing their interpretation of the situation.

Construction of Questionnaire: A **Questionnaire** to be effective must have some essential features. These are:

The size of the Questionnaire should be as modest as possible but not at the cost of necessary information to be collected.

- It should have an elegant appearance.
- As simple as possible.
- Maximum clarity should be maintained.
- Leading questions should be avoided.
- Sequence of questions should be maintained.
- The reliability of the Questionnaire and validity of the questions asked should be maintained.

COMMANDMENTS (16 RULES FOR CONSTRUCTING QUESTIONNAIRE)

Delbert C. Miller in his Handbook of Research Design and Social Measurement provides a guide to the Questionnaire construction.

1. Keep the language pitched to the level of the respondent.
2. Try to pick words that have same meaning for everyone.
3. Avoid long questions.
4. Protect your respondent's ego.
5. Do not assume that your respondent possesses factual information or first hand opinions.
6. Establish the frame of reference you have in mind.
7. In forming a question either suggest all possible alternatives to the respondents or do not suggest any.
8. Avoid ambiguous wording.
9. Give your respondent a chance to express his positive feeling first so that he is not put in an unfavourable light.
10. Decide whether you need a direct question, an indirect question followed by a direct question.
11. Decide whether the question should be open or closed.
12. Decide whether general or specific questions are needed.
13. Avoid biased or leading questions.
14. Phrase questions so that they are not unnecessarily objectionable.
15. Decide whether personal or impersonal questions will obtain the better response.
16. Questions should be limited to a single idea or a single reference.

Questions to be avoided:

- Very Long Questions
- Ambiguous Questions
- Leading Questions
- Complex Questions
- Personal Questions
- Causing Suspicion Questions
- Embrassing Questions
- Irrelevant Questions
- Questions for which answer can be avoided otherwise
- Questions which are likely to yield wrong replies.

Basic Guides to Questionnaire Construction

1. Directions for responding (in planning the Questions it is necessary to consider the directions for answering the questions).

2. Questions to establish favourable respondents rapport.
3. To get the respondent's mind on the topic, to allow the respondents to 'let off steam' and to avoid the respondent's indifference, the questionnaire should carefully formed.
4. Length of the Questions should be short.
5. Design to facilitate tallying procedures.
6. Questions should test the validity of responses.

Merits of Questionnaire Method

- It is very economical.
- The information obtained is of good quality.
- With the help of this method an extensive field may be surveyed and valuable information may be gathered from persons living over a wide area.

Demerits of Questionnaire Method

- It is not easy to break through the pride and prejudices of informants.
- In the case of illiterate people, this method can not be adopted.
- The response from the informants may only be 10% to 15%. Many questionnaires find themselves in waste paper baskets.

A very simple specimen of questionnaire is given below:

A STUDY ON COMPETENCY BASED RECRUITMENT IN SMILE OUT SOURCING IN CHENNAI

1. Name
2. Age ☐ 18-25 ☐ 25-45 ☐ Above 50
3. Educational qualification
   ☐ UG ☐ PG/Professional ☐ Others
4. Gender ☐ Male ☐ Female
5. Marital status ☐ Married ☐ Single
6. Total years of career experience.
   ☐ <1 ☐ 1-5 ☐ 5-10 ☐ >10
7. Years of experience in smile out sourcing.
   ☐ <1 ☐ 1-3 ☐ 3-5 ☐ 5-7 ☐ >7

8. Technical skill in person is of paramount importance while selecting a candidate.

   ☐ Highly agree ☐ Agree ☐ Neutral ☐ Disagree ☐ Highly disagree

9. Assessing the Problem Solving Skills should be a mandatory to select a candidate for any kind of job.

   ☐ Highly agree ☐ Agree ☐ Neutral ☐ Disagree ☐ Highly disagree

10. Interpersonal skills of the candidate are more important than technical skill.

    ☐ Highly agree ☐ Agree ☐ Neutral ☐ Disagree ☐ Highly disagree

11. Communication skill of the employee does play an important assessment criterion for selecting a candidate for any post.

    ☐ Highly agree ☐ Agree ☐ Neutral ☐ Disagree ☐ Highly disagree

12. Competency of a candidate can be best judged by written technical and aptitude tests.

    ☐ Highly agree ☐ Agree ☐ Neutral ☐ Disagree ☐ Highly disagree

13. HR assessment of candidates is necessary for all the levels.

    ☐ Highly agree ☐ Agree ☐ Neutral ☐ Disagree ☐ Highly disagree

14. Positions like supervisors/managers need to be filled with candidates with Man Management Skills.

    ☐ Highly agree ☐ Agree ☐ Neutral ☐ Disagree ☐ Highly disagree

15. A written examination of language will help to test the negotiation skills of the candidates.

    ☐ Highly agree ☐ Agree ☐ Neutral ☐ Disagree ☐ Highly disagree

16. Medical examination should be mandatory while recruiting any employee.

    ☐ Highly agree ☐ Agree ☐ Neutral ☐ Disagree ☐ Highly disagree

17. Stress interview is necessary/useful to assess the stress levels/emotional quotient of the candidate.

    ☐ Highly agree ☐ Agree ☐ Neutral ☐ Disagree ☐ Highly disagree

18. Recommendations, and employee referrals, damage recruitment policy and reputation of the organization.

    ☐ Highly agree ☐ Agree ☐ Neutral ☐ Disagree ☐ Highly disagree

19. Basic computer knowledge is more than enough to recruit the candidate?

    ☐ Highly agree ☐ Agree ☐ Neutral ☐ Disagree ☐ Highly disagree

20. Operating skills can be evaluated by asking the candidate to demonstrate his skill in the particular job.

☐ Highly agree ☐ Agree ☐ Neutral ☐ Disagree ☐ Highly disagree

Techniques to facilitate usable returns:

(i) Covering letter,

(ii) Purpose of the study,

(iii) Guarantee of anonymity or confidentialness of respondents,

(iv) Use of return envelopes and postage; and

(v) Use of participant reply card.

TYPING INSTRUCTIONS

After thoroughly checking the draft of the research report, it should be given for final typing. The different items which are to be considered are paper, margins, indention, spacing between lines and spacing within a sentence.

Paper: The quarto-size white thick un-ruled paper is used for the final printing of the report. The printing should be done on one side only.

Margins: The left margin and the right margin of the report should be 1.5 inch and 1 inch respectively. The top as well as bottom margin should be 1 inch. But, in the pages starting with a chapter, the top margin should be 3 inch.

Indention: The paragraph can be classified into general and indented. The first line of general paragraph is not indented, whereas in indented paragraph, the first line of the paragraph is indented by 10 spaces from the left margin.

Spacing between lines: The entire report should be typed with double spacing except indented paragraphs, tables and footnotes. The indented paragraphs, tables and footnotes are to be typed with single spacing. But there should be double spacing between each neighbouring pair of these single spaced items, that is, between adjacent indented paragraphs as well as adjacent tables.

Triple spacing should be given for the following cases:

- Before each paragraph heading
- Before and after each centre heading, centre subheading, side heading and indented paragraph

Spacing within a sentence: The details of spacing within a sentence are stated below:

Description of item	No. of Spaces
Before and after a slash (/)	0
Before and after a hyphen (-)	0
Between the first quotation mark and the very next word	0
Between the end quotation mark and the immediate preceding word	0
Between the last letter of a word in a sentence and each of comma, Semicolon, colon, exclamation mark, question mark, last parenthesis and last bracket	0
Between words	1
Before the first parenthesis or bracket	1
After a full stop	1
After a comma	1
After a colon	1
After a semicolon	1

ALGORITHMIC RESEARCH REPORT

Algorithm is a sequence of well-defined steps. As per this concept, the main problem is subdivided into meaningful number of sub-problems, then again each sub-problem should be subdivided like this until a well-defined set of steps are obtained to solve the entire main problem. The correctness of the algorithms means the correctness of the logic/steps of the algorithm. Generally, algorithms will have many steps, branching and loops included in different modules. There are problems like layout design, 'Just In Time', production scheduling, line balancing, and portfolio management faced by the research scholar. The solution for each of the above problems can be obtained through algorithms. So, the researcher should come out with newer algorithms or improved algorithms for such problems. For a combinatorial problem, the researcher should attempt to develop an efficient heuristic. The statistical algorithm deconstruct the rating (called raw score) into its various components, and reconstructs the partial scores into underlying factor scores. The degree of correlation between the initial raw score and the final score is called a factor loading. The algorithmic research report can be classified into the following categories:

- Exact algorithmic research report for polynomial problem.
- Algorithmic research report for combinatorial problem.

The main body of algorithmic research report with modelling for combinatorial problem will contain the following:

- Problem identification
- Literature review
- Objectives of the research
- Development of mathematical model
- Design of algorithm (heuristic)
- Experimentation and comparison of the algorithm with the model in terms of solution accuracy.
- Experimentation and comparison of the algorithm with the best existing algorithm (heuristic) in terms of solution accuracy

Exhibit 1

Front page (of a thesis)

A STUDY ON FLOOD FREQUENCY IN THE DISTRICT OF RAMANATHAPURAM (1950 TO 2009)

A thesis submitted to the Department of Economics,
Madurai Kamaraj University, in partial fulfilment of the requirements.
For the award of the degree of Doctor of Philosophy in Economics

By

R. Palani Bava, M.A., M.Phil.

Research Supervisor

A. Mustafa

M.A., (Eco.) M.A. (Hist.), M.A. (Pol.), M.A. (Eng.), M.B.A., Ph.D.,
C.G.T., D.G.T., D.P.D., P.G.D.T., P.G.D.L.L. & A.L.

(University Seal)
School of Economics
Madurai Kamaraj University
Madurai-625021
June 2009

TABLE OF CONTENTS

CHAPTER 9

Scaling Techniques and Interview

INTRODUCTION

Scaling Techniques are the more sophisticated methods to measure the attitudes of respondents. The scaling techniques involve a group of questions of statements in order to provide a more complete view of the respondents' overall attitudes. As C.A. Moser and G. Kalton put it rightly, Scaling methods come into play essential when one wishes to utilise simultaneously a number of observations on each respondent. Scaling techniques are useful in measuring the social behaviour and personality of individuals. It is so also used to measure certain aspects of cultural and social environment.

SPECIFIC PURPOSE OF SCALING

Scaling serves the following specific purposes in social sciences research:

1. Scales help to reduce the complexity of data and present a single score that represent several variables.
2. It helps to test hypothesis by means of quantifying different dimensions of a single underlying concept.
3. It aims at reducing the error in measurement and increasing the reliability of analysis.

TYPES OF SCALES

The scales may be broadly classified into following types:

1. Normal scale
2. Ordinal scale
3. Rating scale
4. Ratio scale
5. Interval scale
6. Factor scaling.

1. Nominal Scale

When the measurement is made with the help of arbitrary number or symbol. It is called Nominal Scale. Nominal scale is simply a system of assigning number or symbol to events in order to label them. The usual example of this is the assignment of numbers of basketball players in order to identify them. A nominal scale is one that consists of more named categories into which objects or individuals are classified. There is an element of arbitrariness in nominal scale. It may be difficult to judge broader-line cases under nominal scale. The scale is not sensitive to various grades within a given category.

2. Ordinal Scale

As ordinal scale contains categories that can be ordered by rank on a continuum, the ordinal scale is used when these is some kind of relationship between two or more classes of objects. For example, if A, B, and C receive leadership scores of 15, 10 and 5 respectively, as an ordinal scale, one may say that A is superior to B and B is superior to C. Indifference curve analysis is the best example of ordinal scale. However, the social science researcher comes across several social phenomena which cannot be simply rank ordered. Moreover, it permits only limited statistical applications.

3. Rating Scale

Compared to the nominal and ordinal scale, the rating scale allows the researcher to interpret not only the order of scale but also the distance between them. Interval scales permit certain mathematical procedures. It can be added or subtracted. The different types of rating are used to judge the persons or objects. They are:

(i) Graphic rating scale
(ii) Itemised rating scale
(iii) Comparative rating scale.

(i) Graphic Rating Scale

This is perhaps the most widely used scale. In this method, the researcher indicates his rating by simply placing a check at the appropriate point on a line that consists of brief statements indicating one extreme of the phenomenon to the other extreme. The scales serves as a guide in locating the rating rather than to provide distinct categories. For example, the following graphic rating scale may be used to enable the student to rate the instructor.

1. Intensely interested in his subject.
2. Definitely interested but not intensely interested.
3. Mildly interested.
4. Rather more disinterested than interested.
5. Definitely bored by the material.

(ii) Itemised Rating Scale

This type of scale consists of a number of statements that are ordered in respect of their scale positions. The scaling expert selects one or two of the categories.

(iii) Comparative Rating Scale

It is used for relative judgement. The position of individual in the rating scale is judged with reference to the position of other individuals or groups with which the individual may be compared. In rank order, the judge is required to rank the individual specifically in relation to one another.

4. Ratio Scale

The highest level of measurement is the ratio scale. A ratio scale includes an absolute zero. It provides usual intervals and gives a rank ordering and it can be used for simple labelling purposes. For example, the variables used in the studies relating to management like the age, income, expenditure, price, market etc. can be measured on ratio scale. It is possible to measure the distance between the grades also.

5. Interval Scale

Compared to nominal and ordinal scale, interval scale allows the researcher to interpret not only the order of scale scores but also the distances between them. It permits certain mathematical procedures.

6. Factor Scaling

Address to the data frame which is multi-dimensional and attempts to uncover underlying dimensions which have not been identified. These scales are designed to inter-correlate items to determine their degree of inter-dependence and thereby give meaning to a set of variables. Osgood's semantic scales are some of the techniques in this category. Though these techniques are versatile, they are still not being widely applied to real business problems.

TECHNIQUES OF SCALE CONSTRUCTION

There are five techniques by which scales are developed. They are:

1. Arbitrary Scaling
2. Consensus Scaling
3. Item Analysis Scaling
4. Cumulative Scaling
5. Factor Scaling.

Arbitrary scales are those that are developed on ad hoc basis and are designed largely through the researcher's own subjective selection of the items. In consensus scaling the selection of statements is made by a panel of judges who evaluate the proposed scale items. In the Item Analysis Scaling, the researcher attempts to measure the response of the respondents to each item with his degree of agreement or disagreement. Summated scales or Likert type of scales are developed by utilizing this type. The usual descriptions for the five categories of Likert scales are:

Strongly Agree	Agree	Uncertain	Disagree	Strongly Disagree

Cumulative scales like differential or summated scales are made up of a series of items with which the respondents indicates agreement or disagreement. The two that are depended on the cumulative approach are:

1. Bogardus scale.
2. Guttman scale.

Factor Scaling

Address to the data frame which is multi-dimensional and attempts to uncover underlying semantic scales are some of the techniques in this category.

Sources of Error in Measurement

1. **Respondent:** The respondent may be reluctant to express strong negative feeling or he may have very little knowledge.
2. **Situation:** Any condition which places a strain on interview can have serious effects on the interviewer – respondent rapport.
3. **Measurer:** Careless mechanical processing may distort the findings. Errors may also creep in because of incorrect coding, faulty tabulation etc.
4. **Instrument:** Error may arise because of defective measuring instrument.

PRINCIPLES OF SCALE CONSTRUCTION

1. **Validity:** A test is valid when it measures what it proposes to measure. This is the most significant criterion in the use of scales. Validity must be appraised with reference to specific situation.
2. **Reliability:** A test or scale is reliable if it consistently yields the same result when repeated measurements are taken of the same subject under the same conditions. Reliability suggests consistency and accuracy from one item to another.
3. **Objectivity:** An objective test or scale is one that produces the same score regardless of who makes it.
4. **Simplicity:** Ease of administration, scoring and interpretation is an important factor in selecting a test, particularly, when expert personnel and adequate budget are not available.
5. **Suitability:** When selecting a scale, one must determine whether the instrument is suitable for the purpose.
6. **Economy:** Tests should save time involved. The expenses in administration is often a significant factor. Particularly if the testing programme is operating on a limited budget.

LIKERT SCALE

The most widely used form of scaling in survey research is Likert scale. It sets up ordinal categories for degrees of agreement, generally including the five levels of Strongly Agree. Disagree, Agree, Strongly Disagree and Do not know. These response categories are attached to a set of statement. Assuming that the responses to each statement are equivalent, you can assign scores of 1 through 5 (or 0 through 4) and create an index by summing up the scores. In respect of negatively worded statements this scoring is reversed. The procedure used to construct a Likert type scale is summarised as follows:

A number of statements believed to be relevant to the attitude being measured are collected and classified either "favourable" or "unfavourable". Items that appear to be neutral are omitted.

A pre-test is conducted in which a group of respondents indicate their opinions of each item according to one of the response categories presented.

Each response is given a numerical score (for example, +2, +1, 0, –1, –2) based on a series of integers in arithmetic sequence. Scores are assigned in such a way that the direction of attitude (favourable to unfavourable) is consistent over all items. For example, if a +2 is assigned to "Strongly agree" for favourable items, the same score is aligned to "strongly disagree" for unfavourable items.

Each respondent's total is obtained by adding his item scores.

Items to be included in the final test are determined by analyzing the results of the pretest. The correlation between statements scores and the total scores is then ascertained. Those statements which have a high correlation with the total scores are then selected for the final test.

The final test is administered to the group or respondents of interest and is scored in the same way as in the pretest. The Likert type scale has certain advantages over the Thurston's differential scale. First, the procedure is such that it is simpler to construct. Second, the Likert-scale provides for expression of intensity of feeling. Third, this scale appears to be more reliable.

Consensus Scaling

The selection of statement is made by a panel of judges who evaluate the proposed scale items. They evaluate the alternatives and determine the level of attitude that the scale item represents. It is popular in sociological space studies than in business research. Thurstone scale is based on this approach.

THURSTONE SCALE

Thurstone scale is one of the earliest and best known forms of scaling. The steps to be followed for the construction of the scale are the following:

First, a large number of statements pertaining to the subject of enquiry are collected. The various methods such as literature survey, personal experience and discussion with knowledgeable persons are followed for developing statements. These statements should range from one extreme of favourable attitude to the other extreme of unfavourable attitude.

Second is the selection of the statements. Thurstone and Chave have given five criteria for selecting the statements. These are: (i) The statements should be brief. (ii) They should be such that it can be accepted or rejected in accordance with the attitude of the respondent. (iii) The acceptance or rejection of the statement should indicate the respondent's attitude. (iv) Ambiguous double-barrelled statements must be avoided. (v) The statements must be related to attitude.

On the basis of the above procedure, the researcher selects some 20 to 30 statements. The scale values are equally spaced. The selected statements are embodied in a questionnaire. They are included in a random order so that there is no hierarchy of scale values. The questionnaire is administered and the respondents with which he agrees. The average of the scale values of all statements he endorses becomes his total scores.

RATING SCALE

Scaling is a method of quantification or measurement. Scaling describes the procedures of assigning numbers to various degrees of opinions, attitudes and other concepts. The rating scale involves qualitative description of a limited member of aspects of a thing or trait of a person. The ratings may be "like or dislike", "above average, below-average" or other classifications with more categories. A few examples are given below:

How for your pain reduced?

(Please √)

Worse than before	No reduction	Good reduction	Excellent reduction

How anxious are you now?

	Very anxious		Slightly anxious		Highly anxious	
Always	Rarely	Neutral		Rarely	Often	Always
My life is worthwhile						My life is not worthwhile

I believe that children should not be forced to study

Strongly disagree	Disagree	Neutral	Agree	Strongly agree

Rating scale may be either graphic scale or an itemized rating scale. The above example are all graphic scales where the rater indicated his rating by a simple tick mark (√) at the appropriate point on a line that runs from one extreme to the other.

This type of rating may sometimes increase the tendency of rater to choose always a particular point (tendency to mark on neutral point). The frame of reference for the researcher and the respondent may vary. This is another limitation.

Itemized rating scale is also known as numerical scale. The researcher attempts to measure the response of the respondent to each item with his degree of agreement or disagreement. Here, a series of statements is presented and the respondents select the statements that are as best reflecting his view or perception or he may order them according to his preferences. The order is progressively in terms of more or less on some property. Here, is an example.

What do you prefer most in your job?

- Leisure time
- Good company policy
- Responsibility
- Independence
- Good wages
- Conducive work atmosphere
- More perks
- Opportunity to use potentials
- Good relationship

This type of scale provides more information to the rater, and increases its reliability. Rating scales are simple. They have wide range of applications. There are three possible errors in Rating scale. They are (a) error of leniency, (b) error of central tendency, and (c) error of hollo effect.

When respondents are too lenient they rate some hardly, it is called error of leniency. They consistently rate strongly agree for almost all the statements.

When the respondents are reluctant to rate. It results in choosing a middle path, i.e., neutral point or least change. This is called error of central tendency.

The error of hollo effect operates when a respondent carries over a generalized bias from one statement to another. For example, a person may rate an individual as beautiful and because of this rating; he may generalize that the person must be smart, intelligent, sociable etc.

Cumulative scales are made up of a series of items with which the respondent indicates agreement or disagreement. Here, the items are related to one another in such a way that an individual who replies favourably to item 1; and one who replies favourably to item 3 also replies favourably to items 1 and 2 and so on. Thus, all individuals who answer a given item favourably should have higher score on the total scale than the individual who answers a given item unfavourably. The two such scales that are depended on this cumulative approach are Bogardus scale and Guttman scale.

INTERVIEW

Interview is another important tool of investigation for a researcher. Interview is the art of eliciting relevant information from a subject who might have been a total stranger until the time of interview. The interview is a method which requires a person known as 'interviewer' asking questions generally in a face to face contact to the other person. Interview is a direct personal investigation. Sometimes, telephone or indirect mass medias may be used to gather information on one to one basis. Interview is the art of eliciting relevant information from a subject who might have been a total stranger until the time of interview.

According to Carter V. Good, interview as a research tool is an oral type of questionnaire or schedule whereby the subject supplies needed information in a face-to-face relationship.

Interview method is always suitable for intensive and confidential investigation. When interview is conducted in an orderly and structured way, it is called structured interview. At other times, the interviews may be unstructured and informal also. The structured interview has predetermined questions and helps the investigator in maintaining the direction of the interview. On the other hand, unstructured interview provides opportunity for the investigator to be more free to explore, change the sequence of enquiry or modify the queries according to the situations.

Unstructured interview does not provide standards for comparability of two interviews. It is more time consuming. The interviewers must be very skillful and be of high caliber and possess deep knowledge in the subject.

In explorative case studies, diagnostic studies, formulative research studies, and specific clinical research methods, unstructured interview is used as a valuable tool for gathering research evidences. On the other hand, in descriptive studies where generalization of observations has to be made on a small sample, structured interview is used as it is being more economical and less time consuming.

Unstructured interview can also be classified as focused interview and non-directive interview. Focused interview is meant to focus attention on the given experience of the respondent and its effects. The interviewer will confine the respondent to a discussion of issues which are relevant.

In the non-direct interview, the interviewer will encourage the respondent to talk about the given topic with a bare minimum of direct questioning.

The interviewer will often acts as a 'catalyst' to a comprehensive expressions of the respondents, feelings and beliefs. This method in widely used in psychotherapy sessions.

Young defines interview as "an effective informal verbal and non-verbal conversation, initiated for specific purposes and focused on certain planned content areas".

Types of Interview

Structured interview, unstructured interview, non-directive interview, directive interview, focused interview, repeated interview, depth interview, individual interview, group interview, etc., are some of the types of interview.

On the basis of purpose: (i) Diagnostic interview (to know the cause of a malady), (ii) Treatment interview (finding the real cause of the malady if it is a psychological case), (iii) Research interview (to gather information), and (iv) Curiosity interview (conducted to satisfy some questions lurking in the mind of a scientist).

On the basis of approach: (i) Non-directive interview (uncontrolled/unguided/unstructured), (ii) Directive interview (structured/guided), (iii) Focused interview (lies in between the directive and non-directive interview), Repeated interview and Depth interview.

The objectives of interview are: (i) To exchange ideas and experiences and (ii) To elicit information.

PERSONAL INTERVIEWS

Personal interview method requires a person known as the interviewer asking questions generally in a face-to-face contact to the other person or persons. The sort of interview may be in the form of direct personal investigation or it may be an indirect oral investigation. In the case of direct personal investigation, the interviewer has to collect the information personally from the sources concerned. He has to be on the spot and has to meet people from whom data have to be collected. This method is particularly suitable for intensive investigation. But in certain cases it may not be possible or worthwhile to contact directly the person concerned or on account of the extensive scope of enquiry, the direct personal investigation technique may not be used. In such cases an indirect oral examination can be conducted under which the interviewer has to cross-examine other persons who are supposed to have knowledge about the problem under investigation and the information, thus, obtained is recorded. Most of the commissions and committees appointed by government to carry on investigations make use of this method.

The method of collecting information through personal interviews is usually carried out in a structured way. Such structured interviews involve the use of a set of predetermined questions and of highly standardized techniques of recording. Thus, the interviewer in a structured interview follows a rigid procedure laid down, asking questions in a form and order prescribed. As against it, the unstructured interviews are characterized by a flexibility of approach to questioning. Unstructured interviews do not follow a system of predetermined questions and standardized techniques of recording information. The interview has relatively greater freedom while recording the responses to include some aspects and exclude others. But this sort of flexibility results in lack of comparability of one interview with another and the analysis of unstructured responses becomes much more difficult and time-consuming than that of the structured responses obtained in case of structured interviews. Unstructured interviews also demand deep knowledge and greater skill on the part of the interviewer. Unstructured interview, however happens to the central technique of collecting information. In case of descriptive studies, we quite often use the technique of structured interview because of its being more economical, providing a safe basis for generalization and requiring relatively lesser skill on the part of the interviewer.

We may as well talk about focused interview, clinical interview and the non-directive interview. Focused interview is meant to focus attention on the given experience of the respondent and its effects. The clinical interview is concerned with broad underlying feelings or motivations or with the course of individual's life experience. In case of non-directive interview, the interviewer's function is simply to encourage the respondent to talk about the given topic with a bare minimum of direct questioning.

Under indirect personal interview, facts are collected by interviewing persons who are directly or indirectly concerned with the subject-matter of the inquiry. Under this method, information is collected from persons who are in possession of such information. The persons are known as witnesses or informants.

Despite the variations in interview-techniques, the major advantages and weakness of personal interviews can be enumerated in a general way. The chief merits of the interview method are as follows:

(i) More information and that too in greater depth can be obtained.

(ii) Interviewer by his own skill can overcome the resistance of the respondents; the interview method can be made to yield an almost perfect sample of the general population.

(iii) There is greater flexibility under this method as the opportunity to restructure questions is always there specially in case of unstructured interviews.

(iv) Observation method can as well as be applied to recording verbal answers to various questions.

(v) Personal information can as well as be obtained easily under this method.

(vi) Samples can be controlled more effectively as there arises no difficulty of the missing returns; non-response generally remains very low.

(vii) This interviewer can usually control which person (a) will answer the questions. This is not possible in mailed questionnaire approach, if so desired, group discussions may also be held.

(viii) The interviewer may catch the informant off-guard and thus, may secure the most spontaneous reactions than would be the case if mailed questionnaire is used.

(ix) The language of the interview can be adopted to the ability or educational level of the person interviewed and as such misinterpretation concerning questions can be avoided.

(x) The interviewer can collect supplementary information about the respondent's personal characteristics and environment which is often of great value in interpreting results.

The interview is superior to the others in the following:

(a) In gaining 'a portrait of personalities', elements of one's character responsible for certain achievements,

(b) In collecting personal data for quantitative purposes, and

(c) In explaing some inexplicable situations.

But there are also certain weaknesses of the interview method. Among the important weaknesses, mention may be made of the following:

(i) It is very expensive method especially when large and widely spread geographical sample is taken.

(ii) There remains the possibility of the bias of interviewer as well as that of the respondent.

(iii) Certain types of respondents such as important officials or executives or people in high income groups may not be easily approachable under this method and to that extent the data may prove inadequate.

(iv) This method is relatively more-time consuming, especially when the sample is large.

(v) The presence of the interviewer on the spot may over stimulate the respondent, sometimes even to the extent that may give imaginary information just to make the interview interesting.

(vi) Under the interview method, the organization required for selecting training and supervising the field-staff is more complex with formidable problems.

(vii) Interviewing at times may also introduce systematic errors.

(viii) Effective interview presupposes proper rapport with respondent that would facilitate free and frank responses. This is often a very difficult requirement.

(ix) If the interviewee is suspicious, sophisticated and ingenious, the interviewer may come back thinking that he has succeeded wonderfully but he might have collected only chaff not grains.

(x) The interview is like diamond exploration; it may succeed beyond one's widest expectations or it may be a sheer flop.

Uncontrolled, unguided and un-structured interview: It does not contain any direct or predetermined question. The interviewer starts the conversation in some way and the interviewee in a free answer-type keeps a flowing conversion. Now and then, the former may delicately direct the flow of talk to relevant facts or events. At the end, the interviewer puts questions for clarification and notes down what he has heard and appears to be pertinent. This kind of interview may be suitable in a case study of say, 'Corruption in State Administration'.

The 'focused interview' is conducted usually with persons, reputed to know the subject of study thoroughly. It proceeds on the basis of a previously prepared interview guide, which indicates in series the significant facets of investigation and which is strictly governed by the hypothesis.

The Board interview is conducted by more than one member of the team. In adopting this method, the choice of a correct venue is important. It may be the respondent's working place, home, a government office, etc.

Group interview: It is undertaken when a batch or group of persons are interviewed together. This saves time and money. But it may lack truth and reliability.

The 'repeated interview' may help to confirm the facts collected in the first round and to gain a full picture of the situation. But it is both expensive and time-consuming.

Short period interview (e.g., opinion and poll surveys).

Prolonged interview (e.g., in-depth studies with little samples relating to the growth and working of TVS company).

Formal (The interview with the Chief Secretary of Tamil Nadu conducted by the CBI).

Informal interview (suited to emotional subjects involving different answers at different times).

For successful implementation of the interview method, interviewers should be carefully selected, trained and briefed. They should be honest, sincere, hardworking, impartial and must possess the technical competence and necessary practical experience. Occasional field checks should be made to ensure that interviews are neither cheating nor deviating from instructions given to them for performing their job efficiently. In addition, some provisions should also be made in advance so that appropriate action may be taken if some of the selected respondents refuse to cooperate or are not available when an interviewer calls upon them.

In fact, interviewing is an art governed by certain scientific principles. Every effect should be made to create friendly atmosphere of trust and confidence so that respondents may feel at case while talking to and discussing with the interviewer. The interviewer must ask questions properly and intelligently and must record the responses accurately and completely. At the same time, the interviewer must answer legitimate question(s) if any asked by the respondent and must clear any doubt that the latter has. The interviewers approach must be friendly, courteous, conventional and unbiased. The interviewer should not show surprise or disapproval of respondent's answer but he must keep the direction of interview in his own hand, discouraging irrelevant conversation and must make all possible effort to keep the respondent on the track.

TELEPHONE INTERVIEW

This method of collecting information consists in contracting respondents on telephone itself. It is not a very widely used method, but plays important in industrial surveys, particularly in developed regions. The chief merits of such a system are:

1. It is more flexible in comparison to mailing method.
2. It is faster than other method.
3. It is cheaper than personal interviewing method.
4. There is higher rate of responses than what we have in mailing method; the non-response is generally very low.
5. Replies can be recorded without causing embarassment to respondents.
6. Interviewer can explain requirements more easily.
7. At times access can be gained to respondents who otherwise cannot be connected for one reason or the other.
8. No field staff is required.

But the system of collecting information is not free from demerits. Some of these may be highlighted.

1. Little time is given to respondents
2. Surveys are restricted to respondents who have telephone facilities.
3. Extensive geographical coverage may get restricted by cost consideration.
4. It is not suitable for intensive surveys where comprehensive answers are required to various questions.
5. Possibility of the bias of the interviewer is relatively more.
6. Questions have to be short and to the point, probes are difficult to handle.

Advantage of Interview

(i) To assess the personality of the respondents it is a very useful tool,

(ii) By means of interview, all information and data needed for the study are collected,

(iii) Delay due to non-responses is avoided, and

(iv) Accuracy of respondents is arrived at by means of asking questions under conducive climate.

Disadvantages of Interview

(i) An interviewer may have bias relating to the socio-economic activities,

(ii) Some-times the interviewer may forget to record the data or he may record irrelevant facts omitting the relevant,

(iii) The chances of controversy are all the great when the interviewer and the interviewee hail from – different social backgrounds with different ideologies and values, and

(iv) Lack of objectivity in approaching the interview is a common drawback of interview. Interviewer and the interviewee are human beings and they are susceptible to the impact of emotions.

Steps Involved in the Interview

1. Planning and preparation.
2. Starting the interview.
3. Asking the questions.
4. Eliciting complete response.
5. Recording the interview.
6. Closing the interview.

Qualities of an Interview

- Honesty,
- Interest,
- Accuracy,
- Adaptability,
- Personality and Temperament,
- Intelligence Education.

Interviewing Errors

With the personal and telephone interview, the interviewer can be a serious source of errors. These errors are related to:

- Interviewer-respondent rapport (interviewers who can establish effective relationships with respondents are able to collect more complete and accurate data),
- Asking the questions (each question in the questionnaire must be read without error or stumbling over words and phrases),
- Repeating the questions and recording responses, and
- Cheating (the personal interviewer who sits at home and fills out the questionnaire is cheating.

CHAPTER

10

Content Analysis

INTRODUCTION

According to Berelson 'Content Analysis (CA) is a research technique for the objective, systematic and quantitative description of the manifest content of communication'. The content analysis should possess the characteristics : (i) objectivity, (ii) system, and (iii) generality. CA is characterized by the fact that the entities analyzed are not usually words but meanings (synonyms or words with similar meanings are grouped in the same category and often include themes or whole phrases).

CA is a method of studying communication. It was developed in the U.S.A. as a branch of social psychology known as 'Communication research'. CA requires the research investigators to use his judgement in making decisions about his data. A content unit refers to a word theme and the like.

CA is not relevant to all documentary research.

It can rarely be used to determine the truth of an assertion or to evaluate the aesthetic qualities of poetry. Moreover, if the analyst uses documents to settle limited issues of fact, such as to determine whether the Indian Express supported Indira Gandhi or Moraji Desai during 1970's, methods other than content analysis could be used more efficiently. The investigator seeks the data from simple factual questions.

CA has been used to assess psychological variables in the context of political decision-making, particularly in the area of foreign policy. The choice of CA is based largely on the inability in most cases to use observational methods to assess the perceptions, attitudes and values of foreign policy leaders at the time of decision. Themes, which are classified into categories such as friendship, hospitality, capabilities, time pressure and alternatives, will serve as the unit of analysis.

Criteria of Good Research Tool

A researcher who is gathering data to test hypothesis must use tools of the investigation appropriately. If the "tool" is wrong, then the evidence cannot be used successfully to test the hypothesis. There are certain important criteria based on which a research tool or instrument is selected for the purpose of study.

They are the reliability and validity of the tools. These two are very essential for effectiveness of data gathering.

Reliability is the degree of consistency that the instrument or procedure demonstrate whatever the tool is measuring. It must measure consistently. Reliability of the data gathered for the research depends on the reliability of the tool used. Whenever a test, questionnaire or inventory is administered repeatedly it must give consistent results.

Validity is that quality of data gathering instrument which enables it to measure what it is supposed to measure. It is also established during the piloting of an instrument. In most cases, it is done simultaneously with procedures to establish reliability. Validity is established through an in-depth review of the instruments, including an examination of the instrument's items to be certain that they are accurately measuring the content or objectives being tested, and by relating scores on the instrument to other measures. Validity may be content validity, sampling validity, and item validity. It may also be criterion-related validity, concurrent validity, and predictive validity.

Reliability is necessary but not sufficient condition for validity. A tool may be reliable but may not be valid.

It is possible through various statistical treatment to establish quantitatively the reliability and validity of the tools. For example, when a researcher states that the psychological tool has a reliability coefficient of 0.70, then he is quantitatively stating that the information obtained is consistent or reliable to the extent of 70% higher the quotient, greater is the consistency.

Similarly when a researcher states that the diagnostic questionnaire has a predictive validity of 0.85, it implies that a diagnosis of disease in the person based on the questionnaire and his chance of getting a disease may be correct to the extent of 85%.

Reliability

Reliable tests are stable in whatever they measure. On the other hand, an unreliable test yields different measurement each time it is applied.

The reliability of an instrument can be expressed in terms of correlation coefficient. There are different types of reliability:

Reliability or stability over time: This is also called as retest reliability. The scores of the subjects correlate high with first and second tests or successive administration of tests.

Reliability or stability over time: Some tests have two or more forms. They may correlate highly.

Stability of items: If scores on certain items in the test are highly correlated with scores on other items, then there is internal consistency or stability. Different statistical procedures are used to measure the internal consistency of the tool.

Stability over scores: Certain psychological tools can be interpreted by two different judges. Two persons can independently score the same set of test papers. When these two sets of scores are highly correlated, then the reliability of the tool is higher.

Standard error of measurement: This is a statistical procedure which permits us to examine whether the given measure is a true measure of a person trait's or qualities. This tells us how much the obtained score differs from the individual's true score. Lesser the difference between the obtained score and true score, greater is the reliability of measurement (scores obtained on the test) Reliability of the testing instrument can be increased by

1. Increasing the number of items of equal quality.
2. Carefully design direction for administration of test.
3. Testing situation must be free from distractions.
4. There should be no boredom and fatigue during the testing situation.

Validity

Basic to the validity of a tool is to measure the right thing or asking right questions. The items of a questionnaire and inventory must appropriately sample a significant aspect of the purpose of the investigation.

Sometimes validity is also thought as utility. There are many kinds of validity depending on the purpose of the tool in the research. They are:

(1) Content Validity,

(2) Construct Validity, and

(3) Criterion related validity (predictive validity and concurrent validity).

Content validity: This refers to the degree to which the tool (test) actually measures or is specifically related to the traits for which it was designed. The examples are as follows:

1. How adequately a test paper measures the knowledge and skills that a student is expected to master in a course of study in a week.
2. How adequately a personality questionnaire purporting to measure jealously has items which indicate jealous feelings, behaviours or statements.
3. How adequately an interest schedule includes statements which elicit information on subjects, likes, and dislikes about profession of job.

Construct validity: This is the degree to which scores on a test can be accounted for by the explanatory constructs of a sound theory Intelligence tests are based on different theories. Hence each intelligence test shows a measures which is appropriate to the theory on which it is based. Construct validity is very important for personality tests. For example, a test measuring Type A personality can be validated by asking the judges to rate the behaviours and gestures of people who score high on the test. The higher rating of the judges and higher scores are found to establish and construct the Type A behaviour.

Predictive validity: Refers to the usefulness of a test in predicting some future performances. For example, a researcher is interested in developing a diagnostic psychological testing tool. For this he wants to discriminate the person for various diseases. Accordingly the tool should be framed in such a way that it scores high for the diseased persons and scores low for the normal persons. In this case the test has a high degree of predictive validity.

Concurrent validity: This refers to the usefulness of a test which is closely relates to other measures (or) scores on another test of known validity. Tests are often validated by comparing their results with a test of known validity. For example, Minnesota Multiphastic Personality Inventory (MMPIT) has been found to be very widely accepted as a valid tool. Many other personality tests which have been developed later have been validated against MMPIT. Many performance tests are validated against paper-pencil tests. Sometimes the researcher can validate the scores on a particular test with that of a rating given by significant relatives of the subject.

A test may be reliable even though it is not valid. Thus, the test can yield scores consistently but of no value. On the other hand, a test which is measuring a specific concept must definitely measure the same concept consistently. This shows that reliability and validity are important criteria for a good research tool. There is also another criterion, practicability. The practicability characteristic of a measuring instrument can be judged in terms of economy, convenience and inexorability: From the operational point of view, the measuring instrument ought to be practical, i.e., it should be economical, convenient and interpretable.

Economy: Tests that can be given in a short period of time are likely to gain the cooperation of the subjects and to conserve the time of all those involved in test administration. The matter of expense of administrating a test is often a significant factor if the testing programme is being operated on a limited budget.

Interest: Tests are interesting and enjoyable help to gain the cooperation of the subject. Those that are dull or seem silly may discourage or antagonize the subject. Under these unfavourable conditions, the tests is not likely to yield useful results.

Interpretation: Test scores and result must be amendable for interpretation by the researchers objectively and uniformly.

DATA PROCESSING

INTRODUCTION

The data that have been collected will be in the form of raw data. The first in analysing the data will be to prepare these data for the type of analysis the researcher plans to carry out. An investigator wants to convert the raw data into numerical equivalents for the purposes of quantitative analyses and statistical testing.

The collected data must undergo some processing before analysis. The objective of processing are the following :

1. Checking the questionnaire and schedules.
2. Reduction of mass data to manageable proportions.
3. Sum up the materials so as to prepare tables, charts and graphs for presenting the results.
4. Minmising the errors.

The processing of data involves activities such as editing, coding and tabulation.

EDITING

Before the data are tabulated and analysis carried, the researcher has to edit the data suitably to make it more meaningful. Editing means inspecting, correcting, and modifying the collected data. Editing is done at the time of collecting the data or later in the central office. Editing the completed questionnaire or schedules is the first and the important stage in the data processing. The scrutiny of interview schedule/questionnaire centres around three main aspects namely: (a) completeness, (b) consistency, and (c) regularity (method of asking questions and recording answers). The following are the usual stages in the editing process:

(i) Initial screening
(ii) Establishing response categories
(iii) Field editing
(iv) Central editing.

Checking and editing the data are needed to see that there is :

(i) Completeness,
(ii) Accuracy, and
(iii) Uniformity.

Completeness

The editor must find whether there is an answer to every question. If the interviewer has forgotten to ask a question or to record the answer, it may be possible to deduce from other data on the questionnaire and fill up the gap.

To overcome this problem tape recorder can be used at the time of interview.

Accuracy

The editor must try to check whether the answers are accurate. Every effort should be made to resolve clear inconsistencies. If this is not possible then the inconsistent entries should be omitted.

Uniformity

The editor must see whether the interviewer have interpreted questions and instructions uniformly.

The investigator has to take into consideration the following basic problems before editing:

(a) Fictitious interviews

(b) Inconsistent replies

(c) Incorrect answers

(d) Incomplete answers

(e) Do not know or no answer.

After a questionnaire is received from the field, it must be inspected to determine whether it is acceptable for use in the study. There must be an editor-in-chief who discusses all problems with the editors and incorporate the changes in the editing instructions.

Coding

After editing is coding or converting the qualitative data in the questionnaire/ schedule to numerical form and presenting it on the coding matrix. The collected data have to be divided into meaningful categories. Coding refers to assigning of number digits or letters or both to various responses so as to enable tabulation of information easy. Goode and Hatt defines coding as 'An operation by which data are organized into classes and number of symbol is given to each item according to the class in which it falls.' According to M. Parton, 'Coding consists in assigning a number of symbol to each answer which falls in a predetermined class.' For example, the coding can be done for the following multiple choices of the given question:

How do you spend your leisure time?

Reading books	1
Playing outdoor games	2
Visiting friends	3
Attending domestic work	4
Watching TV	5
Any other specify	6

The following four major rules guide the establishment of category sets. Categories should be:

Appropriate to the research problem: Generally 3 to 5 categories are considered reasonable. For example, categorisation of respondents on the basis of age, say under 20 years, 20 to 30 years, 30 to 40 years and above 40 years may be relevant to the study.

Exhaustive: There must be a category for every item. For example, there is a question in the questionnaire 'What is your favourite form of entertainment?'

The alternatives will be:

1. Movies
2. Skipping
3. Boating
4. Watching TV
5. Other (describe).

Mutually Exclusive: In an occupational survey, the classification of respondents may be professional, managerial, sales, clerical, craftsman, operatives and unemployed.

Single Dimension: Every class in the category set is defined in terms of one concept. In the example cited above, a respondent is both a salesman and unemployed. The 'salesman' label expresses the concept of occupational type while the response 'unemployed' is another dimension.

Computer Coding: There are now computer cards, tapes, disketts into which information are coded. Accuracy and sophisticated calculations are the benefits of using computers in the processing of data. Computerisation of data makes the tabulation easy and precise.

Code Sheets: Code sheets instruct the coders how to handle each question. When codes are defined, a listing of all types of responses being assigned to each code should be made on the code sheet. The code sheet consists of the following elements:

(a) **Heading:** The heading identifies the study.

(b) **Column identification:** Each applicable columns is to be listed on the left-hand side of the page.

(c) **Coding instructions:** Limitations/restrictions and required multiple codes are to be stated next to each code where applicable.

(d) **Special instructions:** Instructions for the use of 'borrowed columns'.

Analysis and Interpretation of Data

Analysis and interpretation are giving meaning to the collected information by comparing them with the existing information. For example, a survey undertaken in Madurai shows that the per capita income in Madurai in 2008 was say Rs. 4,000. This information is not useful. It can be associated with the income of the other cities.

Analysis is placing the collected data in some order or format, so that the data acquire a meaning. Interpretation involves drawing conclusions from the gathered data.

1. *Procudure for Analysis*

There are three tasks to be performed if the collected data are to be used in the most effective manner:

(i) An intensive review must be made of all the data collected.

(ii) These data are then analysed with the help of techniques selected earlier.

(iii) The results emerging from these analyses are then related to the study's hypotheses and objectives.

The collected data have to be analyzed fully. For example, a large soap manufacturer made a study of market trend for his two brands namely A and B. The researcher collected data regarding sale of these two projects for the year 2000 and 2001. On the basis of the data collected, an analysis has been made. The analysis, thus, made is not relevant since it has not been taken into account the total bleach sales for the industry, the activities of the competitors and the causes for the decline in sales.

There are numerous articles published in various trade and academic journals describing new models and techniques for analysis. Besides, text-books on statistics outline various analytical techniques. These documents should be consulted before deciding the frame work of analysis.

The analysis may be descriptive analysis and casual analysis.

2. *Descriptive Analysis (One Dimensional Analysis)*

Descriptive analysis is largely the study of distribution of one variable. This analysis shows the benchmark data and measures the state or condition at any particular time. This analysis is the prelude to bivariate and multivariate analysis.

Table 10.1: Birth Rate* in India

Preiod	Birth rate per 1000
1961 – 71	41.2
1971 – 81	37.2
1981 – 91	32.5
2000	28.0
2005	23.8
2008	22.1

*Birth rate indicates the number of live births occurring during the year, per 1,000 population estimated at mid-year.

3. *Bivariate Analysis*

The bivariate analysis is placing the collected data into tabular form, so that the real meaning of these data can be derived. The starting point of Bivariate Analysis is to develop simple dimensional data. Then put the data into two, or more categories. This analysis is explained with the help of a survey. A study was undertaken among Madurai City residents to determine their movie-going habits. A sample of 1,000 persons was randomly interviewed. Out of 1000 sample members 267 (26.70 per cent) are regular movie goers and 733 (73.30

per cent) are not regular movie goers. These facts are given in the following table:

Table 10.2: Movie Attendance Among Sample Residents

Category	Number	Percentage
Regular Movie Goers	267	26.70
Not Regular Movie Goers	733	73.30
Total	1000	100.00

4. *Sequential Analysis*

The data presented in a table reveals one factor at a time. This analysis is called sequential analysis. A further analysis of the data regarding movie goers showed that the college students were more frequent movie goers than non-college students.

Table 10.3: Students in Terms of Movie Attendance

Category	College Students	Non-college Students	Total
Regular Movie Goers	130 (37%)	137 (21%)	267
Not Regular Movie Goers	220 (63%)	513 (79%)	733
Total	350 (100%)	650 (100%)	1000

The data presented in the above tables reveal one factor at the time.

5. *Casual Analysis*

This analysis explains how one variable affects another. We may analyse to find out whether two variables (dependent and independent) are related or not. There are different ways which we might determine whether such correlations do exist or not.

A researcher is usually interested in understanding why sales are larger in some markets than in others. Sales are affected by product quality, advertising, price or other things which can be controlled by the manager. The variable is such as sales. Sales can be dependent variable. Changes in brand's price, package and advertising may affect the brand's sales. These variables are called independent variables.

The cross tabulation, correlation and regression analysis are methods of analysis which can explain why there are different variations in a dependent variable. The casual analyses are done with the help of statistical tools.

INTERPRETATION

Interpretation means drawing inferences from the collected facts after the analytical study. According to C. William Emory interpretation has two major aspects namely establishing continuity in research through linking the results of a given study with those of another and the establishment of some relationship with the collected data.

Interpretation helps the researcher to understand the abstract principle that works beneath his findings. Interpretation enables the researcher to establish concepts, which will be the basis for future research. Moreover, interpretation helps the target audience to understand the real significance of his research findings.

Pre-requisities of interpretation

(i) The data should be homogeneous.
(ii) The data should be adequate.
(iii) The data should be appropriate.
(iv) The data should be scientifically analysed.

TECHNIQUE OF INTERPRETATION

(i) **Relationship between variables**: The basic objects of every analytical research is to find out the relationship between any two variables. There may be three types of relationship:

(i) Symmetrical relationship
(ii) Reciprocal relationship
(iii) Asymmetrical relationship.

The interpretation of data can be made with the help of these relationships.

(ii) **Percentages:** Percentage are used in making comparison between two or more series of data. They are also used to describe the relationships. They are also used to describe the relationships. The following tables shows the uses of percentages.

Table 10.4: Sales of Two Types of Cars in Tamil Nadu

Cities in Tamil Nadu	Maruti	Per Cent	Fiat	Per Cent
Chennai	300	30	400	20
Madurai	200	20	500	15
Coimbatore	200	20	500	25
Tiruchirapalli	150	15	350	17.5
Tirunelveli	150	15	450	22.5
Total	1000	100	2200	100

With the help of the above table it is easy to compare the sales of cars in different cities of Tamil Nadu.

(iii) **Average:** The mean, median and mode are commonly used. Instead of using long statistical tables, the use of average makes the interpretation very simple.

(iv) **Dispersion:** Dispersion refers to the amount or the magnitude of the spread. Measures of dispersion include range, inter quartile range, average deviation and standard deviation. These measures help to interpret the data more scientifically.

3. Precautions in Interpretation

Correct interpretation requires a high degree of skill, care, judgement and objectivity on the part of the researcher.

(i) **Adequate data:** The data should be large and unbiased. Then only the results will represent the Universe.

(ii) **Variation in definition:** Variations in definition make the comparisons inappropriate. For example, while comparing the national income figures of two countries, say, India and U.K., it is essential to find out whether the definition for National Income in both countries is the same. If the definition is different in the two countries, then the comparison is not possible.

(iii) **Errors in the use of statistical tools:** The use of inappropriate statistical techniques, inadequate sample size and faulty calculations make the result spurious.

SOCIOMETRIC MEASUREMENT

Some 15 years ago, and about 15 years after the appearance of the earliest Bogardus scale, J.L. Moreno and Helen Hall Jennings applied a measure of social distance which differed radically from the Bogardus approach. The chief divergence of this method, usually called sociometry, from the earlier technique lies in the fact that it is concerned with attractions and repulsions between individuals with a small group and with the group structure as defined in these terms. Helen Jennings has described this method as follows:

"Stated briefly, sociometric may be described as a means of presenting simply and graphically entire structure of relations existing at a given time among members of a given group. The major lines of communication, or pattern of attraction and rejection in its full scope, are made readily comprehensive at a glance".

The technique has been applied in such widely diversified situations as informal groups, school classes, prisons and other organizations, and industry. Since there is considerable latitude in the application of sociometry, it may be well to begin with a consideration of an early statement of its characteristics made by Jennings in 1943:

"The form of the sociometry test as applied up to the present has had three characteristics:

1. "A specific number of choices is allowed, varying according to the size of the group tested;
2. "A specific criterion for choice is used, varying with the functional activity of the group...."
3. "Different levels of preferences are designed for each choice".

As an example of this type of sociometry procedure, a study referred to earlier has been selected. This is a volume dealing with the technique of studying school classes, and the requirements above are met in terms of this situation. Three choices were allowed for each child, and the situation was defined as one in which the criterion for selecting other children in the class was "liking to work with them on a study committee". The levels of choices were designated by asking the children to designate with the number 1 child they would most like, their second choice with 2, and their third choice with 3.

The major point to note here is the fact of designated choice situation in such a way as to be meaningful – in this case by asking the children to name others with whom they would like to do committee work. Obviously, there is an infinite number of ways in which the situation can be structured. For example, in an institution it might be: "With whom would you like to eat, share a room spend your leisure, etc.?" Or industry with whom would you like to work – play – visit, etc.?" The important thing here is (1) that the situation must be a real one to the group being tested. And also (2) that it must fit the sort of sociometric structure which is being studied.

To return to the study of the school children, the next step is tabulation of the data.

Another method of analysis, however, employs the sociogram. The function of this diagram is to make clear the network of acceptance and rejections in a graphic way.

The sociogram also offers other possible methods of analysis. Since each child shows a different frequency of being chosen and further a different frequency of the level at which he is chosen, there exists the possibility of scaling the individuals as to "acceptability". This, in turn, implies the possibility of scaling on the basis of willingness to accept others because of the limitation to only three choices. However, the method is not well suited to this approach. An example of a variant of this method suited to such an analysis is found on the Ohio State Social Acceptance Scale. It will be noted that instead of a series of choices of children, each child is rated on a friendship scale. Thus, if these results are put into a matrix, every cell will have an entry. The total row at the bottom will, then, show the relative position of each child in the class in terms of being accepted. In this case, there is also the possibility of a total column which would contain the sum of the ratings given by each child.

These techniques have recently been given increasing application in practical situations, such as administering children's camps, choosing members of flight crews and the recent Army inauguration of the "buddy system". They have also been of great utility in introducing new knowledge and techniques in underdeveloped regions, for they aid in ascertaining the channels of power, gossip, and communication within a small village, a rural area, or a larger geographical region.

These and other variants of sociometric technique offer rather simple methods of ranking individuals on a continuum of "acceptability" or "outgoingness" on the part of group members, where their use is justified, they may be powerful research tools, since they meet the general problems of scaling very well.

A. Definition of the continuum: The existence of a social-distance continuum can be accepted only in so far as it proves valid by other criteria. There seems no trouble in defining the continuum in these scales as social distance, however, as long as the stimulus, i.e., the choosing situation, is appropriate to the conclusions drawn.

B. Reliability: This type of scale is suitable only for test, re-test, and reliability measurement. Jennings, however, givens ample evidence that "choice position" is slow to change and that sociometric measurement may therefore, be considered reliable.

C. Validity: In the same volume, the findings indicate that the independent criterion of case studies and behaviour observation provide satisfactory indicators of the validity of sociometric tests.

DEDUCTION

Deduction is a logical process in which specialized conclusions are drawn from general propositions. The deductive method is also known as 'abstract', 'aprioristic' or 'axiomatic' method. In this, major premise (or general proposition assuming an air of universal truth) is the real core of knowledge; for example, take the premise 'men are mortal' and the special inference 'Socrates was mortal'. The inference hardly adds anything to the existing fund of knowledge. Suppose the major premise is wrong as in 'all sheep are carnivorous' and its reference 'Mary's little lamb is also carnivorous and it will eat mice and frog'.

The conclusion is as much false as the major premise. Before using any major premise in deductive analysis, the researcher should check up whether it is correct under all circumstances.

The classical economist used the deductive method. Adam Smith's system of free economic enterprise culminating capitalism is based on two major premises namely, man is actuated by self-interest and Laissey faire policy. To quote his famous example, 'it is not from the benevolence of the butcher, the browser and the baker that we expect our dinner, but from their regard to their own interest'. Secondly, 'every man has an instinct to barter and exchange'. Each individual thus specialises in that occupation for which he has the greatest aptitude and exchange what he produces for goods he wants. Malthusian theory of population is based on the proposition, 'every human being is dominated by the instinct to procreate'. Because of the passion between the sexes, population increases in geometric progression (unless checked by artificial methods). Man is a social animal; this is s major premise in political theory of the state. Generally, the major premises in the deductive analysis adopted by the social scientists are universal truths.

Induction

Inductive method proceeds from the particular facts to general conclusions. These conclusions shed some light and human knowledge is extended in inductive method. In the inductive method, conclusions shed some light and human knowledge is extended. Ernest Engel's study of the family budgets of the working classes was indeed confined to a small sample of 50 families. But his inductive reasoning and conclusion that expenditure on food varies inversely with the family income is broader in its coverage than the small sample from which it is derived. Thus, inductive reasoning illuminates and may be fruitful, yet, it is at times hazardous. There can be no certainty that its conclusions would be true and hold good always. According to Galbraith, the modern giant corporations do not aim at maximizing profit. It is true in the cases he cites. But from his premises, it would be rash and wrong to generalize that profit maximization is dead and not the major objective of any firm in may country. Inductive reasoning is a valuable tool, but it needs to be handled with extreme caution. It's use calls for deliberation and correct judgement based on rich experience.

Qualities of Inductive Reasoning

The following qualities of inductive reasoning have to be considered by every researcher:

(i) The conclusions hold only in terms of probabilities, never with certainty. A leap in the dark is always involved when we apply conclusions to cases not yet observed.

(ii) Since no comprehensive account of all the circumstances that bear upon an inductive argument is ever possible, one who accepts the conclusions of inductive reasoning places dependence on the personal discernment and integrity of the persons making the observations and completing the argument. "The priceless ingredient of every induction is the honour and integrity of its maker. It is less dangerous to have a scoundrel among deductively reasoning mathematicians than to have a scoundrel among statisticians.

(iii) We must assume that there exists some uniformity in the system of facts to which the premises and the conclusions of inductive reasoning relate. That is the rational justification for the leap in the dark which it involves.

Scientific generalizations are based on two methods known as induction and deduction. Induction is a process of reasoning from particular cases to whole group of cases, from specific instances to general rules. Deduction on the other hand is a process of reasoning from general to particular, from given premises to necessary conclusions. Both the methods are interdependent and hold an equally important place in any scientific analysis.

When hypothesis is formed we use deductive reasoning as we try to form certain generalization from the broad theory itself to be made applicable to certain hypothetical conditions. In order to test the hypothesis we have to collect data, analyze it and draw conclusions from it. It involves an inductive process. After a theory has been involved it is tried on special cases for its validity and the researcher has to utilize the deductive process again.

Then through out the scientific research the researcher has to use sometimes alternately and at times even simultaneously both inductive and deductive methods of reasoning. According to Charles Beared – "It would be interesting to find an assumption premise that is not in some way entangled with experience and method of inference from particulars". The following remark of Prof. Marshall corroborates with this statement. "Induction and deduction are both needed for scientific study as right and left foot for working".

Difficulties of Logical Methods

The logical methods described above are subject to two difficulties, viz. (1) plurality of causes and (2) inter mixture of effects.

1. **Plurality of causes:** A phenomenon is not the result of one single cause. At times it may be caused by number of factors. If it so, discovery of a particu-

lar cause becomes a difficult task. To take an example, a rise in the prices may be caused by a number of factors opening together. It would, therefore, be difficult to locate the particular causes and their contribution in the creation of the phenomena under the study. Plurality of causes requires a large number of cases to be studied before the correct inference can be drawn.

2. **Inter-mixture of effects:** Just as an incident may be caused by a number of causes, in the same way one single causative factor may produce a number of results. The various effects may be so mixed up together that it may be quite difficult to sort them out.

Cluster Analysis: It is a classification method that is used to arrange a set of cases into clusters. It is the name given to a diverse collection of techniques that can be used to classify objects individuals, quadrats and species. The aim is to establish a set of clusters such that cases within a cluster are more similar to each other than they are to cases in other clusters. The classification has the effect of reducing the dimensionality of a data table by reducing the number of rows (cases). The classification will depend upon the particular method used. This is because it is possible to measure similarity and dissimilarity in a number of ways. Large number of calculations are needed which can put a heavy demand on the computer.

Factor Analysis: There are two approaches to factor analysis,- 'principal component analysis' (the total variance in the data is considered) and 'common factor analysis' (the common variance is considered). Factor analysis is an interdependence technique. The complete set of interdependent relationships are examined. There is no specification of either dependent variables, independent variables, or causality. It is originated in psychometrics, and is used in social sciences, product management, marketing operations research and other applied sciences that deal with large quantities of data. It is a statistical technique used to explain variability among observed random variables in terms of fewer unobserved random variables called factors. The observed variables are modeled as linear combinations of the factors, plus 'error' terms. Factor analysis assume that all the rating data on different attributes can be reduced down to a few important dimensions. This reduction is possible because the attributes are relate. The rating given to any one attribute is partially the result of the influence of other attributes. If we want to build testable model to explain the intercorrelations among input variables, we should carry out a factor analysis.

Common factor analysis: It involves a testable model. Under this model, unique variables are required to be uncorrelated. Components are not latent variables. They are linear combinations of the input variables and thus determinate. Factors, on the other hand, are latent variables, which are indeterminate.

Principal component analysis: It does not involve a testable model. Here, residuals are correlated. If our goal is to fit the variances of input variables for the purpose of data reduction, we should carry out principal components analysis. The use of principal components in a semantic space can vary somewhat because the components may only 'predict' but not 'map' to the vector space. This produces a statistical principal component use where the most salient words or themes represent the preferred basis.

Merits of Factor Analysis:

- There is flexibility in naming and using dimensions.
- Both objective and subjective attributes can be used.
- It is based on direct inputs from customers.
- It is fairly easy to do, inexpensive, and accurate.

However, usefulness depends on the researchers ability to develop a complete and accurate set of product attributes. If important attributes are missed the procedure is valueless.

Discriminant Analysis: It may have a descriptive or a predictive objective. It may be used for two objectives either we want to assess the adequacy of classification, given the group memberships of the objects under study, or we wish to assign object to one of a number of (known) groups of objects. In marketing discriminant analysis is a statistical technique for analyzing data. It is applicable when there is only one dependent variable but multiple independent variables (similar to ANOVA and regression analysis). It is similar to factor analysis in that both look for underlying dimensions in responses given to questions about product attributes. It is different from factor analysis in that it is not an interdependence technique: a distinction between independent variables and dependent variables (also called criterion variables) must be made. It also differs from factor analysis in that it builds these underlying dimensions based on differences rather than similarities.

Methods of Discriminant Analysis

(i) **K-NNs Method:** Non-parametric (distribution-free) methods dispense with the need for assumptions regarding the probability density function. They have become very popular especially in the image processing area. The K- NNs Discriminant Analysis assigns an object of unknown affiliation to the group to which the majority of its K neaeest neighbours belongs.

(ii) **MDA method:** Multiple Discriminant Analysis adopts a similar perspective to PCA (Principle Components Analysis), the rows of the data matrix to be examined constitute points in a multidimensional space. So also do the group means vectors. Discriminating axes are determined in this space in such a way that optimal separation of the predefined groups is attained.

(iii) **Linear Discriminant Analysis:** It is the 2-group case of MDA. It optimally separates two groups, using the Mahalanobis metric or generalized distance. It also gives the same linear separating decision surface as Bayesian maximum likelihood discrimination in the case of equal class covariance matrices.

ADVANTAGES OF DISCRIMINANT ANALYSIS

1. It is noted for its analytical simplicity and computational possibility.
2. MDA is most appropriately used for feature selection.
3. Linear discrimination is most widely used in practice.
4. The k-NN rule is simply defined and implemented, especially if there is insufficient data to adequately define sample means and covariance matrices.
5. It is possible to focus on the variables used in order to investigate the differences between groups, to create synthetic variables which improve the grouping ability of the data, to arrive at a similar objective by discarding irrelevant variables, or to determine the most parsimonious variables for graphical representational purposes.

   However, there is no best discrimination method.

REFERENCES

1. Dhingra, H.L. Diversification In Indian Manufacturing Industries. Punjab University, 1968, Supervisor: T. N. Kapur.
2. Ackoff, Russell, L.: The Design of Social Research, Chicago, University of Chicago Press.
3. Bailey, Kenneth, D.: Methods of Social Research, New York.
4. Bowley, A.L.: Elements of Statistics, 6th ed. London, P.S. King and Staples Ltd.
5. Beveridge, W.I.: The Art of Scientific Investigation, New York, Vintage Books.
6. Cochran, W.G.: Sampling Technique, New York.
7. Dasgupta, Sugata: Methodology of Social Science Research, New Delhi.
8. Goode, William, J., and Hatt K. : Methods in Social Research, New York, McGraw-Hill.

9. Kothari, C.R.: Research Methodology – Methods and Techniques, New Age International Publishers, New Delhi.
10. Lundberg, G.A.: Social Research: A study in Methods of gathering data, Newyork.
11. Marguerite G. Lodico, Dean T. Spaulding and Katherine H. Voegtle: Methods in Educational Research: From Theory to Practice, Jossey-Bass, A Wiley Imprint, San Francisco.
12. Pande, G.C.: Research Methodology in Social Sciences, 1989, Anmol Publications, New Delhi.
13. Pauline Young: Scientific Social Surveys and Research, Prentice Hall Inc.
14. Webb, Sidney and Beatrice: Methods of Social Study, London, Longmans.
15. Rao, K.V.: Research Methodology in Commerce and Management.

Solved Problems

1. STUDENT'S 't' TEST

A machinist is making engine parts with axle-diameters of 0.700 inch. A random sample of 10 parts shows a mean diameter of 0.742 inch with a S.D. of 0.040 inch. Compute the statistic you–would use to test whether the work is meeting the specification.

Solution :

Here the sample size $n = 10$

Hence, the sample is small sample.

Also the sample mean $\bar{x} = 0.742$ inches

and the population mean $\mu = 0.700$ inches are given.

S.D. $= 0.040$ inches

∴ We use Students 't' test

Null Hypothesis H_0 = The product is conforming to specification

Alternative Hypothesis = $H_1 : \mu \neq 0.700$

The test statistic is,
$$t = \frac{\bar{x} - \mu}{\frac{S.D.}{\sqrt{n-1}}}$$

Here $\bar{x} = 0.742$ inches, $\mu = 0.700$ inches

S.D. = 0.040 inches and n = 10

$$\text{Degree of freedom (d.f.)} = n - 1 = 10 - 1 = 9$$

$$\therefore \quad t = \frac{0.742 - 0.700}{\frac{0.040}{\sqrt{10-1}}} = \frac{0.0742 - 0.700}{\frac{0.040}{3}}$$

$$= \frac{0.742 - 0.700}{0.0133} = \frac{0.042}{0.0133} = 3.15$$

∴ The calculated value of $t = 3.15$

The table value of t at 5% level with 9 degree of freedom.

$$t_{0.05} = 2.26$$

Since the calculated value of t > tabulated value of t, H_0 is rejected.

∴ The product is not meeting the specification.

2. F-TEST

In one sample of 8 observations that sum of the squares of deviations of the sample values from the sample mean was 84.4 and in the other sample of 10 observations it was 102.6. Test whether this difference is significant at 5% level.

Solution :

Here $n_1 = 8, \quad n_2 = 10$

Also, $\Sigma(x - \bar{x})^2 = 84.4 \quad ; \quad \Sigma(y - \bar{y})^2 = 102.6$

$$Sx^2 = \frac{1}{n_{1-1}} \quad ; \quad \Sigma(x - \bar{x})^2 = \frac{84.4}{7} = 12.057$$

$$Sy^2 = \frac{1}{n_{2-1}} \quad ; \quad \Sigma(y - \bar{y})^2 = \frac{102.6}{9} = 11.4$$

Null Hypothesis $H_0 = S^2x = S^2y$

Now $F = \frac{S^2x}{S^2y} = \frac{12.057}{11.4} = 1.057$

i.e., Calculated $F = 1.057$.

Tabulated value of Fat 5% level for (7, 9) degrees of freedom is 3.29

i.e., $F_{0.05}\ (7, 9) = 3.29$

Since calculated F < tabulated F.

We accept the null hypothesis.

3. CHI-SQUARE TEST

A sample analysis of examination results of 500 students was made. It was found that 220 students had failed, 170 had secured a third class, 90 were placed in second class and 20 got a first class. Do these figures commensurate with the general examination result which is the ratio of 4:3:2:1 for the various categories respectively.

Solution :

Null Hypothesis H_0 : The observed results commensurate with the general examination results. Expected frequencies are in the ratio of 4:3:2:1

Total frequency = 500 $\Rightarrow$ 4 + 3 + 2 + 1 = 10

500/10 = 50

If we divide the total frequency 500 in the ratio 4:3:2:1 we get the expected frequencies as 200, 150, 100, 50

(50 × 4 50 × 3 50 × 2 50 × 1)

Class	Observed Frequency (0)	Expected Frequency (E)	0 – E	$\frac{(0-E)^2}{E}$
Failed	220	200	20	2.000
Third	170	150	20	2.667
Second	90	100	– 10	1.000
First	20	50	– 30	1.000
	500	**500**		**23.667**

Calculated $\chi^2 = \frac{\Sigma(0-E)^2}{E}$

$= 23.667$

$= n - 1$

Degrees of freedom $= 4 - 1$

$= 3$

$\chi^2_{0.05} = 7.81$

i.e., tabulated value of χ^2 at 5% level for 3 d.f. = 7.81

Since calculated $\chi^2_{0.05}$ > tabulated $\chi^2_{0.05}$

We reject the null hypothesis i.e., the observed results are not commensurate with the general examination results.

4. H-TEST

The following are the final examination of marks of three groups of students who were taught computer by three different methods:

First method : 94, 88, 91, 74, 87, 97

Second method : 85, 82, 79, 84, 61, 72, 80

Third method : 89, 67, 72, 76, 69

Use the H-test at the 0.05 level of significance to test the null hypothesis that the three methods are equally affective.

Solution :

1. Setting up of Hypothesis

   Null hypothesis = $H_0 = \mu_1 = \mu_2 = \mu_3$

   Alternative hypothesis : $H_1 : \mu_1, \mu_2, \mu_3$ not all equal.

2. Level of Significance : Here = $\propto$ = 0.05

3. Calculation of test statistic = Ranking the data jointly from 1 to 8, we find that

$$R_1 = 6 + 13 + 14 + 16 + 17 + 18 = 84$$

$$R_2 = 1 + 4.5 + 8 + 9 + 10 + 10 = 55.5$$

$$R_3 = 2 + 3 + 4.5 + 7 + 15 = 31.5$$

($\therefore$ there is only one tie and tied marks are each designed the rank 5.5)

Also

$$N_1 = 6, \qquad N_2 = 7, \qquad N_3 = 5$$

$$N = N_1 + N_2 + N_3 = 6 + 7 + 5 = 18$$

$\therefore$ Test Statistic :

$$H = \frac{12}{N(N+1)}\left(\frac{R_1^2}{N_1} + \frac{R_1^2}{N_2} + \frac{R_1^2}{N_3}\right) - 3(N+1)$$

$$H = \frac{12}{18 \times 19}\left(\frac{(84)^2}{6} + \frac{(55.5)^2}{7} + \frac{(31.5)^2}{5}\right) - 3 \times 19$$

$$H = \frac{2}{57}\left(1176 + \frac{3080.25}{7} + \frac{992.25}{5}\right) - 57$$

$$H = \frac{2}{57}(1176 + 440.04 + 198.45) - 57$$

$$H = \frac{2}{57} \times 1814.49 - 57$$

$$= 53.67 - 57 = 6.67$$

Degrees of freedom = k − 1

= 3 − 1

= 2

$\therefore$ χ^2 (for 2 d.f. and $\propto$ = 0.05) = 5.991

Division : Since H = 6.67 exceeds

$\therefore$ $\chi^2_{0.05}$, 2 = 5.991 (from χ^2 table)

So the null hypothesis is rejected.

We conclude that the there methods are not equally effective.

Index

I

J

K

L

M

Q

R

S

T

U

V

W

Y

NOTES

NOTES

NOTES